new S

Living Among Meat Eaters

The Sexual Politics of Meat:
A Feminist-Vegetarian Critical Theory

Neither Man Nor Beast:
Feminism and the Defense of Animals

Woman-Battering

The Inner Art of Vegetarianism:
Spiritual Practices for Body and Soul

The Inner Art of Vegetarianism Workbook

Meditations on the Inner Art of Vegetarianism

Journey to Gameland: How to Make a Boardgame
from Your Favorite Children's Book
(WITH BEN BUCHANAN AND SUSAN ALLISON)

EDITOR OF

Ecofeminism and the Sacred

Animals and Women: Feminist Theoretical Explorations
(WITH JOSEPHINE DONOVAN)

Violence Against Women and Children: A Christian Theological
Sourcebook
(WITH MARIE FORTUNE)

Beyond Animal Rights: A Feminist Caring Ethic for the Treatment
of Animals
(WITH JOSEPHINE DONOVAN)

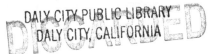
Living Among Meat Eaters

THE VEGETARIAN'S
SURVIVAL HANDBOOK

Carol J. Adams

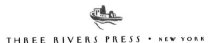
THREE RIVERS PRESS • NEW YORK

S

The "flow and control chart" on page 41 is reprinted from *The Inner Art of Vegetarianism Workbook* (New York: Lantern Books, 2001), p. 84. Suggestions for experiencing the meditative qualities of cooking on pages 221–22 are from *The Inner Art of Vegetarianism* (New York: Lantern Books, 2000), p. 152. Used by permission of the publisher. The "Vegetarian Patrons of Restaurants" card in Appendix C, used by permission of the Vegetarian Foundation. The "International Vegetarian Card" in Appendix D, used by permission of the Physicians Committee for Responsible Medicine.

Published by Three Rivers Press, New York, New York. Member of the Crown Publishing Group.

Random House, Inc. New York, Toronto, London, Sydney, Auckland
www.randomhouse.com

THREE RIVERS PRESS is a registered trademark and the Three Rivers Press colophon is a trademark of Random House, Inc.
Printed in the United States of America

DESIGN BY DEBORAH KERNER

Library of Congress Cataloging-in-Publication Data

Adams, Carol J.
     Living among meat eaters: the vegetarian's survival handbook / Carol J. Adams.—
1st ed.
        p.   cm.
     Includes bibliographical references.
        1. Vegetarian cookery.   I. Title.

TX837 .A29 2001
641.5'636–dc21

                                                                                            2001027760

ISBN 0-609-80743-9
10   9   8   7   6   5   4   3   2   1
First Edition

For Douglas and Benjamin,
the next generation—
may they live abundantly among vegetarians

Contents

Contents

The symbolism of meat-eating is never neutral.

To himself, the meat-eater seems to be eating life.

To the vegetarian, he seems to be eating death.

There is a kind of gestalt-shift between

the two positions which makes it hard to change,

and hard to raise questions on the matter

at all without becoming embattled.

—Mary Midgley

Living Among Meat Eaters

1

When Worlds Collide

We all live among meat eaters. When I was a meat eater, I never thought about this fact. Once I became a vegetarian, it was inescapable. If nothing else, popular culture reminds us at every turn:

> Eat low on the food chain. Barbecue a vegetarian.
> —BUMPER STICKER IN TEXAS

> Screw vegetarians.
> —POSTCARD FROM OREGON

> Vegetarians Not Welcome.
> —BILLBOARD AT THE BORDER TO SOUTH DAKOTA, MID-1990S

> VEGETARIANS WELCOME . . . to watch us eat steak.
> —A MINNESOTA STEAK HOUSE

> I didn't fight my way to the top of the food chain to be a vegetarian!
> —BUMPER STICKER IN CALIFORNIA

> Horrifying Vegetarians Since 1980.
> —RECURRING AD IN THE NEW YORK TIMES FOR A STEAK HOUSE

> I like animals. They're delicious.
>
> —BUMPER STICKER IN NEW YORK

Because meat eaters are in our lives, we are in theirs. And then what happens? Our worlds collide.

Here are stories of collisions from vegetarians around the country:

"Just before Thanksgiving, I was having a conversation with a meat eater. When he learned I was a vegetarian he said, 'So I guess you don't celebrate Thanksgiving.' "

"Once I was forced to eat at a barbecue/grill/steak house. Of course, I was doubtful going in, but I consoled myself with the assumption that most such places sport a salad bar. The funniest part was a chalkboard sign at the entrance advertising that the vegetable of the day was . . . 'Chicken and dumplings!!!' Yow. I knew I was in trouble at that point. Still I forged ahead, but to my dismay I found that nearly every item at the salad bar (except the iceberg lettuce) contained meat in some form or another— 'for flavoring.' Oh well."

"I adopted a turkey from Farm Sanctuary for Thanksgiving, and my mother and brother were trying to figure out how to get that particular bird on the Thanksgiving table to thwart my efforts."

"When I explained to someone why I was a vegetarian, he said, 'If we don't kill the cows, they will die.' "

"Two years ago when my father died, I went back to the small town in rural southern Indiana for the funeral. The neighbors had a potluck dinner for the family after the services and there was not one dish without meat or by-product! Even the wilted lettuce salad had bacon grease. I ended up going to the local sub shop for a veggie sandwich. I was upset, but didn't say anything since the neighbors were trying to be helpful. In the middle of cow country where all meals have meat

and potatoes, people just don't seem to realize it is possible to live without meat."

"They simply don't understand that I don't miss meat and I'd probably drop dead if I ate it. I'm not missing out on anything. I never get the urge to go have a closet Big Mac. I get very defensive when someone gives me a knowing grin and says, 'A little meat won't hurt you, just try some, it's really gooood.'"

"A woman I met recently would not eat popcorn that I offered her as she said it was part of a violent process when the chemical reactions occur to make it pop. She then turned around and ate meat for lunch."

"I pointed out a comparison of [the] water required to yield one pound of beef versus one pound of vegetables to my father, a GP. He replied, 'Paranoid, neurotic.'"

"Someone introduced me as 'Paige, she's vegan.' And the woman I was introduced to asked, 'Where's Vega?'"

When we are meat eaters living among meat eaters, our world is reflected back to us, confirming our choices. When we become vegetarians, we stop being reflections; we may even be accused of breaking the mirror.

"Meat eaters always ask with derision whether or not I'm associated with PETA; they think that my food looks unappetizing; one fellow likened my alfalfa sprouts to 'shaving my Chia Pet.'"

"'What do you eat, salad?' Grrr. . . . I can't understand why what I eat (or don't) seems to bother people so much. I'm like a novelty at work. The vegetarian. I can't argue my point of view without getting into an unwanted debate, trying to justify myself."

"I feel like bonking people over the head sometimes when they say, 'What do you eat?' especially because when I start in with my recipes for various Indian, Italian, and other dishes they quickly change the topic. They wanted the question to be rhetorical. One friend asked me this same question repeatedly, and clearly didn't give a damn what my answer was! She seemed more bent on convincing herself that vegetarianism would be impractical than on observing the patience necessary to think about it. I almost wanted to say, 'Oh, cardboard boxes and aluminum cans.'"

"I am sixteen and ever since I turned vegetarian four years ago, I have not gotten much support from my peers. In fact, when I told a good friend of mine, she became extremely defensive. The next day she had written the following on her backpack: 'We were not put at the top of the food chain to eat vegetables.' I wasn't terribly hurt by the comment or anything, but [by] the fact that she had been fine with all the other oddities of my character, except for this one. I was now introduced as 'Erika . . . the vegetarian,' accompanied by the rolling of her eyes in a sarcastic manner. I suppose things are better than when my mother was in college and people called her a communist for her vegetarianism."

Just when we think our work is done, we discover that it has only begun: the challenge isn't *becoming* a vegetarian; it is *being* a vegetarian.

"When I was thirteen and newly vegetarian, a friend of my parents offered me tortellini salad, saying it was vegetarian. And after I had eaten it he laughed as if he had played a marvelous trick on me and told me the tortellini was filled with veal. I don't know still if it really was. But I am still shocked that an adult could derive joy from 'playing' that sort of trick on a child."

"Every time I visit a friend in California, she goes through a great fuss to be sure she's hidden all the meat. She also makes a big fuss *about how difficult it is to feed me, and how worried she is that I won't get enough to eat. She never forgets to tell me about her vegetarian aunt, who lived to be well over ninety but, supposedly, always had a lot of gas."*

"When I flew home from France, the airline did not get my request for a vegan meal, and all they had was chicken or steak. I explained to the flight attendant that I do not eat meat, and asked if I could have the vegan sidedishes. She was nice, but then another attendant told me that chicken was not meat, and when I said that it came from an animal, he insisted that chicken is vegetarian. He would not give me the sides unless I took the chicken, but finally the other flight attendant told him it was my choice."

Once we stop eating meat for whatever reason, the meat-eating world seems less welcoming. Plenty of books exist that tell you how to become a vegetarian.★ This book discusses how to relate to others after you have taken that advice. This book is not about diet; it is about self-understanding and interpersonal relationships.

THE PROBLEM

When my son was in second grade, the discussion one week focused on nutrition. The children were handed a chart about the food groups provided by the American Dairy Association. One of the charts was called the "meat group." Depicted on this page, besides various forms of meat, were images of tofu and peanut butter. The discussion about the "meat group" began.

★In this book, I presume that I am speaking both to vegetarians and vegans. At times I address issues specific to vegans. Many vegetarians find that their concerns about the suffering of animals and about their own personal health motivate an adoption of an animal-free or plant-based vegetarianism. See my book *The Inner Art of Vegetarianism: Spiritual Practices for Body and Soul* for my discussion of my own progression and suggestions for becoming a vegan. In terms of living among meat eaters, however, this book is addressed to all vegetarians, because anyone who stops eating dead flesh can trigger the types of reactions from meat eaters that are discussed in the following pages.

After a while, Douglas stated that he did not eat meat.

Another child exclaimed, "But I would die if I didn't eat meat."

At home, Douglas described that day's interaction. He told of the child who exclaimed, "But I would die if I didn't eat meat." Looking at us, concerned for that boy's confusion, he said, "But I don't eat meat and I'm not dead."

This is the gestalt shift that Mary Midgley describes in the epigraph to this book: meat eaters and vegetarians see the others' diet completely differently. We see the meat eaters' food as death (the death of the animals especially); they see it as life-giving—they get nourishment from it. In fact, to extend Midgley's insight: we see our diet as a choice of life (whether it is our own, healthier life, the life of the animals, or the life of the planet); meat eaters see our diet as death (if not actually death, as this second-grader feared, then the death of traditions, of pleasure as they know it, of their control over food choices).

When adults ask, "How do you survive as a vegetarian?" they are asking two questions at once: survive meaning, 1) How do you "make do?" and 2) Can you really *survive* on that food? To take away meat may not mean literal death, but it implies to them the loss of everything associated with the pleasures of eating. To them, our diet is one of scarcity, limitation, loss, deprivation; and their diet is one of abundance, choice, enjoyment. This is the gestalt shift. More than anything else, this explains the oft-heard exclamation, "I'd *die* without a hamburger."

How you live your vegetarian life can become a challenge because of this conflict in meaning—we see death in their meals, they see it in ours. Attempts will be made to disempower your viewpoint. Your diet is the issue, but you become the target.

Imagine that the gestalt shift is like the shifting of the tectonic plates when an earthquake occurs. An intense amount of energy is released; and the world is changed. Sometimes after an earthquake, we have to rebuild. So, too, with the gestalt shift.

To you, your vegetarianism is a natural progression in eating habits and philosophy. To nonvegetarians, it represents a profound disjunction. Most meat eaters experience it as a judgment on them as well, and get defensive. Vegetarians sigh and say to themselves, Here we go again.

I asked vegetarians to send me their pet peeves about meat eaters. What a lengthy list I compiled! A recurring "peeve" was that meat eaters experience our vegetarianism as a judgment on them:

Vegetarians' Pet Peeve: Defensiveness

"People take my culinary decisions so personally!"

"People apologizing to me for eating meat."

"Meat eaters who ask me why I am a vegetarian and, when I tell them, accuse me of preaching, proselytizing, judging them."

"When they make rude comments that make others laugh and are hard to recover from without being rude yourself. You feel alienated and attacked. You also feel their stupidity and are tempted to lash out at it."

"I find that most of the time people try to disgust me by making stupid comments like 'So you're a vegetarian. . . . So I guess a nice piece of animal flesh is out of the question.' I find this totally absurd and rude. What are they trying to prove? I don't try to force my opinion on anyone, and I don't criticize their choices, and I expect the same respect for mine."

"I haaaaaaate when people challenge me about it, because in no way am I forcing my opinions on everyone, so why should they force theirs on me?"

"I spend twice as much time defending my diet as eating it."

In the category of frustrating interactions, the question "How do you survive?" and its variations was a close second:

"People who ask, 'What do you eat?'"

"The @#$%! protein myth."

"Trying to convince my father that I'm not going to die."

"People who think I eat fish."

"People who ask, 'But do you eat animal crackers?'"

Another set of pet peeves was organized around the fact that we vegetarians become an easy target. This shows up in so many ways:

"People who blame my diet if I get ill. If I'm sick it must be because I'm a vegetarian. If I'm tired it must be because I'm a vegetarian."

"You are afraid to give any bad impressions, because everyone you meet will tell somebody else, 'I met a vegan once. She seemed weary and unhappy to me.' They'll conveniently forget that you just ran two blocks to catch a school bus that left early."

"Being teased at many a meal."

"When someone heard I am vegetarian, he said, 'Oh, what about your husband. Is he normal?'"

"Being looked at as a freak or extremist."

Meat eaters, seeing themselves as the normal ones, often throw curveballs at you, trying to bring you back into the meat-eating world:

"Having my grandmother call me long-distance from her deathbed, asking me to please eat . . . *MEAT LOAF*!"

"Meat eaters who try to bring me back into the fold."

"Meat eaters who want to talk sense into me."

"People purposefully not disclosing nonvegan food contents to get me to 'try' something."

"People who try to get me to eat meat."

Meat eaters seem clueless at times about what your life-giving foods are. Consequently, the frustrations of actually eating with meat eaters are many:

"Being told, 'You can pick the meat off.'"

"People who don't understand that I won't 'pick the meat out.'"

"Being duped about what is in the food."

"Having someone tell me a dish does not contain meat and it does, and then they say, 'Oh, that little bit of meat doesn't matter.'"

"My family insists on calling Gardenburgers 'Stinkyburgers.'"

"People who say about a restaurant, 'Oh, it's okay. They have a salad bar.'"

"When the table is full of people and I'm asked in front of everyone why I don't eat meat."

"Relatives who bring foods like Kentucky Fried Chicken when I invite them over for a meal."

Little things and daily frustrations often remind us of the conflict in meaning that organizes our world. The world is structured for meat eaters:

"There's a 'meat' compartment in every refrigerator."

"Microsoft Word redlines *veganism*." [Microsoft Word speller doesn't have "vegan" in its dictionary.]

"It's not easy to find a vegan friend."

Finally, there is simply the olfactory problem. Many vegetarians reported that they were discomforted by "the smell of meat" and "the smell of meat eaters."

What do these pet peeves reveal about living among meat eaters?

Many of the interactions that were reported violated trust. It is natural to expect that we can take others at their word—that they are not going to serve us meat or mislead us about meat. Yet vegetarians continually report that they cannot trust this to be so, as the person who was given veal tortellini discovered. Some meat eaters, and maybe it's just a few—but vegetarians all around the world keep encountering those few!—are willing to lie and dissemble to ensure that your diet is the same as theirs.

These pet peeves also tell us that many meat eaters don't listen to you. You define vegetarianism, and yet they offer you fish. You say you are happy and yet you are encouraged to try something "just this time."

Additionally, these interactions reveal the rigidity of some meat eaters. They cannot welcome change. Even from a deathbed, a grandmother reaches out in concern about vegetarianism. At a more mundane level, we experience this rigidity when we are asked, "What will it do to Thanksgiving?" or, even more profoundly, it is assumed we can't observe Thanksgiving at all if a (dead) turkey is absent.

These pet peeves also tell us that there is something more going on than simply repetitive interpersonal reactions. They reveal that meat eaters feel that your change in diet is about them. They read themselves into your dietary choices.

For, in fact, becoming a vegetarian often reveals more about your friends, family, and society at large, than it does about yourself. Why? You changed. They didn't.

Now, I know that some vegetarians have not experienced these frustrations and that some meat eaters are always gracious, loving, and accepting of another's vegetarianism. Great. No problem. For those who do not experience the dramas revealed in the list of pet peeves, I say, "Hurrah!" This book was written for those not so lucky: those who have stopped eating meat or wish to stop eating meat, and live among difficult meat eaters. I know that both groups—frustrated vegetarians and frustrating meat eaters—exist. Ever since the publication of my book *The Sexual Politics of Meat,* I have been hearing from them. A few years ago, I decided to invite vegetarians to write to me specifically about their experiences living among meat eaters. I was surprised, and saddened, by the answers, often poignant, to one specific question: "What was your best experience interacting with meat eaters?"

Three responses recurred. The first one was "I have had no good experiences with meat eaters." Many of them reported on exhausting discussions that became debates. Repeatedly I was told:

"I have no tales of inspiration."
"I don't know of any."
"I have yet to have an amusing/inspiring incident happen with
    a tableful of meat eaters."
"I'm scared to eat with friends sometimes."

The second response revealed that, for many vegetarians, a good experience with meat eaters is merely the absence of criticism, not the presence of acceptance. They reported, "I call a good experience one in which I am not picked on for being a vegetarian." This is a minimal standard at best, and I discovered it being applied in various situations:

"I was on a date with a meat eater, and he didn't ridicule me
    for not eating meat."
"The most successful time I had eating with a meat eater was
    when I happened to be fasting."
"Our friend thought that the local Chinese buffet restaurant
    was now making sushi. What he actually ate was the raw
    chicken cut up for the barbecue table."

The third response revealed that the positive could be experienced. It centered on stories about sharing vegetarian food. Repeatedly I encountered variations on this statement: "My best experiences are around the food I eat and prepare for others":

"When they like my meal better than theirs. Mine is cheaper
    and healthier."
"A meat-eating friend who calls often just to ask what I'm
    making for dinner."
"Cooking a meal for meat eaters and they never missed
    the meat."

"'Converting' a meat eater."

"Getting served a preordered veggie plate at an expensive wedding, and all the meat eaters were jealous of it."

"When I finally got my father to try tofu. Granted, it did take a heart attack to get my father to start eating a more vegetarian-based diet. . . ."

This third set of responses proves a point we often forget: show, don't tell.

Living Among Meat Eaters wants to transform your experiences from the negative to the positive. Why should you be burdened with meat eating—albeit someone else's—when you have stopped eating meat? I want to raise our standards for interactions: a good experience is not just the absence of a bad experience. But how do we change these relationships when we often feel powerless in the face of what meat eaters are doing, both in their eating patterns and their behavior toward us?

Well, it is easier than you think. Change your perspective. A meat eater's reaction to a vegetarian often has less to do with the vegetarian and much more to do with the meat eater. You don't need to shoulder someone else's burden. There is something affirmative you can do instead. You have the power to keep the worlds from colliding. All you need are some elemental navigational skills.

THE ANSWER

Simply put, the thesis of this book is that *you should see every meat eater as a blocked vegetarian.* Despite knowing at some level that plant-based vegetarianism is better for them, meat eaters have decided not to change. Something is keeping them blocked, and whatever it is assumes more importance than the pull of vegetarianism. This blocking force will be present in their relationships with vegetarians. Meat eaters teach us what their issues are. They are daily showing us what is blocking them.

Yes, it is hard at times to live with a decision that separates us from our friends, family, and co-workers. Even harder, though, is realizing that one does not need to be a meat eater and then failing to do anything about it. After all, meat eaters live among meat eaters, too. We may feel excluded from meals centered around meat. They face a different problem, the omnipresence of meat. Meat-centered assumptions about meals drown them in opportunities to eat meat. The words that explain our vegetarianism, which to us express freedom, joy, relief, happiness are heard as pronouncing judgment on them for being blocked. We are happy, but we are heard as angry. They don't want to be reminded about meat eating because it reminds them of their unfinished work.

Vegetarians remind meat eaters that they are blocked. What is blocking them are issues specific to them. Simply by being a vegetarian, you will most likely trigger those issues that are blocking them. Consequently, meat eaters' interactions with you announce the symptoms of their blockage. Meat eaters project their own uneasiness on vegetarians. If they accuse you of judging them, that is because they are judging themselves. If they sabotage you, that is because they are sabotaging themselves. By recognizing that the issues they bring to interactions with us represent their own inner conflicts—inner crises that preexist these interactions—we can respond better in terms of our own peace of mind, and also in terms of theirs. We can say to ourselves, "This person has a problem with my vegetarianism. It is their problem, not mine."

People have many explanations for eating meat; vegetarians have heard all of them. If their explanations sound hollow, it may be because they are. For some people, their predicament is not so much that they choose to eat meat as that they have chosen not to change. As a result, interactions are often really about the nature of change—or, more precisely, not changing. We are drawn into the meat eater's drama of being blocked. And what do blocked vegetarians do? They spend more energy antagonizing, interrogating, criticizing, fearing, and belittling us than dealing with themselves. This is the best way for them to stay blocked.

A liberating approach to living among meat eaters is available to each of us: recognize them as *blocked* vegetarians, but relate to them as *potential* vegetarians. As a result, we reorient our own goals in any interaction: it is not to defend our diet but to help them remove the defensiveness encircling theirs. This means that you have to be alert to what they are keeping hidden from themselves. Relate to them on a deeper level by finding ways to keep them from setting the agenda. Their agenda is, most often, to stay blocked.

The Benefits of This Approach

Something happens—a confrontation, a conflict, a disturbance, an unpleasant interaction. "What just happened?" we ask. "And why?"

Often the first answer that comes to mind is "This interaction is about *me*. It is about my vegetarianism." We offer an explanation that focuses on us, keeping it personal, and thus take the interaction personally. "It happened because of something I did." If we keep the explanation at the personal level, we will not understand. It is not solely because of who we are.

Or we answer the question by saying, "This happened because of the relationship I have with X. We just can't talk about this." If we keep the explanation at the interpersonal—"It was because of who X is and how X and I interact"—we will still not understand what just happened. The only way we can understand "what just happened" is through the systemic approach this book provides. Our culture produces blocked vegetarians, and our interactions with meat eaters are a result of that. So, we say to ourselves, "This happened because our culture has caused this individual to be a blocked vegetarian." With this systemic approach, we ourselves are removed from the equation.

A systemic approach offers several benefits. First, these interactions are not about you. So try not to take them personally or explain them by focusing on yourself. No longer situated in the realm of the personal, the interactions can be objectified. Second, this approach gives you the opportunity to be prepared. Third, an interpretative framework provides you with tools for responding. Ordinarily you experience the push and pull of these daily interactions; now you are the one who has *leverage*. This gives you choices among a range of responses or non-responses. You do not have to be the one who is moved, thrown off course, by an event. Instead, you can be the mover.

I don't assume that you want to change meat eaters into vegetarians (though many meat eaters, being blocked, project this motive on you). I do assume that you would like to move through the meat-eating world with more ease. That is what this book offers: the opportunity to gain some control over difficult situations.

For those of you who do wish to convert meat eaters—I've got some news. The methods we often choose to convince meat eaters of the appropriateness of our diet instead convince them that they would never want to adopt it. That is because we send nonverbal as well as verbal messages.

Several fronts exist when meat eaters and vegetarians interact. Meat eaters keep us focused on their arguments. This front is often the *least* important one. We have to become equipped to read social interactions. Here are the basic guidelines for doing so:

Guidelines for Living Among Meat Eaters

- View meat eaters as blocked vegetarians and their reactions to you as their symptoms of being blocked. When something happens, tell yourself, "This is happening because meat eaters are blocked vegetarians. What shall I do? I have the choice to respond or not to respond."
- Be at peace with your vegetarianism and help others see that you are at peace with your diet.
- The closer the relationship (family, lover, roommate), the more likely that dietary differences will bear the burden of many nondietary conflicts. Watch out!
- Nonvegetarians are perfectly happy eating vegan meals, as long as they are unaware that they are doing so.

- Living among meat eaters is a lot like living with adolescents: *don't take things personally;* their outsized reactions are ways of trying to level the playing field.
- Be patient. Assume everyone can become unblocked.

Viewing meat eaters as blocked vegetarians changes the nature of our responses. At times, this means we must cultivate the art of not responding. It also means that we must develop the ability to work with blocked energy. Finally, it requires recognizing that people who are blocked cannot take care of our needs; theirs overwhelm them so. Thus, it is essential for you to be prepared to take care of yourself.

On the one hand, I am saying there is a simple solution to meat eater–vegetarian relationships—consider all meat eaters blocked vegetarians. On the other hand, I am saying something more: once we recognize this we have to acquire certain skills. *Living Among Meat Eaters* offers these skills. They are easy to adopt and they will immediately change the dynamics that have deprived you of the ease of living as a vegetarian. They start with essential rules of thumb:

Rules of Thumb for Living Among Meat Eaters

- Assume your needs will not be met in any meat-eating context—airplanes, foreign countries, private homes, restaurants. Always have a backup plan when eating out.
- Don't let any rudeness spoil your experiences. Respond to offensive behavior courteously, according to the rules of etiquette, and move on.
- You have the right not to answer questions you are asked and to stop a conversation that makes you feel uneasy.
- Don't talk about your vegetarianism at a meal if people are eating meat. Learn the art of deflecting attention.
- Volunteer to bring something whenever you are invited somewhere.
- Channel negative energy to the positive. The constellation

of negative emotions associated with blocked meat eaters—denial, guilt, defensiveness—can dissolve in the presence of positive energy. As one vegetarian explains, "I love hearing the word 'vegetarian' from the lips of those who are not! They are rehearsing for the future!"

- Remember that following a vegetarian diet is always an affirmation of wholeness. Bring that sense of wholeness to your interactions with meat eaters.

I know that my recommendations often seem to run counter to our desires. I am basically asking vegetarians to exhibit a moral, emotional, and spiritual maturity that is quite demanding. And yet it is as worthwhile as it is demanding. Moreover, this approach works! If what I recommend seems hard and perhaps even unfair, because I am asking vegetarians to be the mature ones in their relationships with meat eaters, please trust me! All of that hardship is outweighed by the benefits you will acquire. You will be able to move through the meat-eating world with a sense of freedom and less conflict.

If everyone is a blocked vegetarian, then what we experience in our culture and in our interactions isn't the "meat-eating world" as much as it is immense blocked energy surrounding vegetarianism. We have confused the two. *Their* world is hurtling toward us because of the gravitational force of *our* world. But they don't need to collide.

Because of the intensity of the gravitational force, we are drawn into the meat eater's drama of being blocked. But we don't have to be. We do not have to feel, "Here we go again!" Instead we can say, "I know what is going on and I know how to respond." Often this involves simply stepping out of the way. In the pages that follow, I'll tell you how to do so.

2

Are You at Peace?

Meat eaters want to know if you are at peace with your diet. They won't ask you this directly. They ask, "But don't you miss meat?" They mean, "Are you at peace with giving up meat?"

If you are at peace, maybe they, too, could be at peace living without meat.

> If you are not at peace, why should they try?
> Are you at peace?
> If you are, how do you communicate that sense of peace?
> If you aren't, what is needed to discover a sense of peace?

It has been suggested that only two main story plots exist: a journey is undertaken, or a stranger comes to town. When you stop eating meat, you are both the person who goes on a journey and the stranger who comes to town. The journey is the decision to stop eating meat and the steps you take to change your diet. Through this process, you become a stranger to family, friends, and co-workers, because you are no longer like them.

They want the old familiar "you" back. How they experience this new "strange" you may influence whether they themselves set out on the journey. They are watching you.

Yes, people are studying you. They want to know that vegetarianism has improved our lives, not just our health. Have we shrunken in spirit because we are anxious about food? Are we more argumentative, even if it is because nonvegetarians draw us into a debate and do not want to drop the issue? If we are embittered, they think, Why bother? Our diet is being judged by how we relate to others and to food. Has our journey made us more open, happier, relaxed, at peace, or have we returned tired, cranky, and, as with many journeys, complaining about the food we were served?

It does not matter to them that it may be difficult to be at peace living without meat in a meat-eating world, among them. It does not matter to them that after the journey we are feeling hungry, alienated, depressed, bitter, excluded. What matters is, are you at peace with your journey? Vegetarians who are not at peace with their vegetarianism represent meat eaters' worst fears, not their best hopes and dreams.

OUR JOURNEY

To become vegetarians, we undertook an inner journey, a journey that required unpacking rather than packing. We decided what we could live without. Could we live without meat? At first we might have *hoped* that the answer was yes; soon we *knew* the answer was yes. Along the way we probably discovered many aspects of ourselves that we did not know.

Any journey is disruptive of everyday life. This journey is no different. We disrupt whatever relations with our family, friends, and ethnic group that are consolidated by traditions of eating meat foods. You soon discover how meat eating at times mediated your relationships not only with family members but with your heritage and your family's expectations about that heritage. People may feel personally rejected if you don't eat meat and if you don't participate in the local or ethnic traditions.

When we journey away from meat eating, we know where we are heading. We may be equipped with marvelous guidebooks explaining how to undertake the journey. But what do we know of the destination itself? Until it is realized, it is an idea only. We know what we are giving up—familiar tastes and the comfort of a diet shared by so many of our acquaintances and family. But we don't know what it feels like to arrive, to be a "vegetarian." Will we miss meat? How will we handle the day-to-day demands of this new diet? Beginning our journey, we know this absolute truth: One cannot be a vegetarian in imagination or desire alone. Consciousness and act must be united. A journey requires leaving home.

Facing Our Fears

In order to take our journey, we had to prevail over our fears about leaving home and its comfortable familiarity. In avoiding their own journey, meat eaters have permitted these fears to have legitimacy in their lives.

People then bring their own fears to their interactions with you. If we are at peace with our diet, we can be a sign of reassurance that these fears can be dealt with. If we are not at peace with these issues, then they will have confirmed, at a nonverbal level, that their fears are legitimate.

Fears Meat Eaters Have

Clearly, one fear meat eaters have is that they will have to forgo one of their few pleasures in life. Most people today feel very stressed and quite unhappy. They have few things to look forward to, and these are almost always sensual pleasures. Take away their favorite foods, and life has that much less to offer them. Tasty food gives them one of their few reasons for putting up with life's many unpleasant struggles. This is a major fear, but not the only one:

- They fear separation, a break in relationships with friends and family, of disrupting the family or inner circle.
- They fear being different, and being judged for that.

- They fear calling attention to themselves.
- They fear the unknown.
- They may have a fear of new foods (such a person is called a "neophobe").
- They fear that their appetite will not be satisfied: "I'll miss the meat." "I'll be hungry." "I won't like the food." "I won't enjoy the taste of vegetarian food."
- They fear that they will endanger their health rather than improve it: "I'll get sick." "I won't get enough protein."
- They fear confronting a negative experience: the loss of security and enjoyment and identity of being a meat eater.
- They fear losing the feeling of comfort, the comforts associated with eating meat, including a sense of being taken care of, of being a "child" in relationship to a parent.
- They fear that they or their background will be judged.
- They fear realizing that their culture and their parents betrayed them by telling them, "Meat is good for you."
- They fear losing their sense of humor.
- They fear becoming like vegetarians they already know.
- They fear losing the power and control associated symbolically with eating meat.
- They fear that they'll lose their cynicism. They might discover they do care.
- They fear that "my life will no longer feel abundant."

We who have returned from the journey—changed, as journeys tend to change us—have a degree of wisdom about these fears that entrap others. Facing our fears, what we have learned is that fears don't have to frighten us. We have found ourselves on the other side of them.

We discovered that some of those fears were simply the games the mind plays upon us as it clings to an old self, the comfort of the past, and a fixed identity. We had to acknowledge what our fears were and to examine them.

We also discovered that some of those fears were legitimate. We *did* feel some of the things we feared feeling. But in the process, we learned something more important: it was okay to experience those feelings. One can live without meat *despite* having these feelings. "Hello, discomfort; hello, craving; hello, awkwardness. I feared I would feel you, and I do. Here you are again. But it's okay. This journey is more important to me than letting you limit my sense of possibility." It takes courage to acknowledge that fear exists yet still do what one feels is necessary. Acting despite fears does not eliminate them; it just puts them in their place.

Meat eaters fear the emotional effort required by being a vegetarian. When we are at peace, we communicate the ease of being a vegetarian.

Meat eaters fear living with uncomfortable feelings; they fear that their desire for meat will no longer be satisfied and this does not, to them, seem bearable. They don't understand that homesickness is a natural part of traveling. It is okay to have that feeling of missing meat. It is okay to have the feeling of desire for meat foods. It is even okay to feel regret at times. At that time, we talk to others for support, or choose a vegetarian comfort food, or write in our journal, or whatever it is we have developed as a tactic to balance those feelings with the freedom of being who we are now. What meat eaters don't realize is that the worldview that includes vegetarianism can offer the kind of joy they fear they will lose if they give up meat.

We who have stopped eating meat know that there are worse things than those seemingly unbearable feelings. What would be worse for us would be to have remained at home because we feared homesickness. Then we would be living with the sense of failing our own best intentions or intuitions. Furthermore, meat eaters are living with uncomfortable feelings right now. They are simply *familiar* uncomfortable feelings.

What we learn when we face our fears is that fears don't have to frighten us, immobilize us, keep us from moving. Now we have the wisdom and confidence that comes from facing our fears.

But other things may be keeping us from being at peace with our vegetarianism. Yes, meat eaters may reveal their symptoms of being blocked. But there is also the possibility that though we are unblocked, we are not symptomless. Interactions with meat eaters may trigger feelings in us. If you need to be recognized, or you need to be taken care of, and you go out to eat and there is nothing for you to eat, your neediness can be triggered. No one has recognized your vegetarianism, and no one has taken care of you. These are needs you have regardless of whether you are a vegetarian or not. But now your vegetarianism triggers them. We have to be prepared to recognize our own neediness and ensure that vegetarianism does not accentuate it.

Vegetarianism, while enacting our best hopes for ourselves, may also arouse or raise some of our deepest insecurities. If you were uptight about food, your anxiety may now be more pronounced. If you weren't, you may become so. If you have always had a sense of feeling left out, issues of meat eating and vegetarianism in mixed company may arouse those feelings. If you already feel neglected in relationships, that meat eaters may neglect your food needs will touch you more deeply. If you feel you aren't listened to, this will be magnified if you try to explain your decisions about vegetarianism and nobody wants to listen to you. If you are already argumentative, debates with meat eaters may become ferocious expressions. Few people really want to watch their friends' home movies of their vacation trip. Not having it together is like showing a travelogue no one wants to see. Moreover, it reinforces meat eaters' fears that vegetarianism, regardless of its claims, really doesn't improve people's lives. It leaves them lessened, reduced, diminished.

The Fear of Scarcity

One particular fear circles around many an interaction between meat eater and vegetarian.

"What do you eat?"

"What's left to eat?"

"So, do you only eat plants?"

Or, as one man in Austin, Texas, yelled out his car window at activists for a vegan Thanksgiving: "What do you want us to eat, *vegetables*?"

Meaning: "How can you accept diminishment of food choices?"

Meaning: "Are you at peace eating just those few foods? Because I certainly wouldn't be! I want to feel abundance in my life! How can your life be abundant?"

Their question is not really "Can it be done?" but "Will it diminish my life?"

The epigraph to this book identified a gestalt shift: we see death; they see life. Conversely, we see life in our plant-based diet; they see death—the death of pleasure and enjoyment. They see deprivation and scarcity where we see abundance. We answer their questions about what we eat by declaring, "There is plenty of good food for us to eat!"

But, often, in interacting with meat eaters, they encounter us in places where that assertion is clearly not true. We might be at a restaurant (that they picked!) and nothing is available for us. Whatever the situation, the emotional tension around food—needing a sense of its abundance—spills over into the interaction. People not only want to feel nurtured, they want to be sated—jumbo meals, groaning buffets, triple burgers, all appeal to this desire to be fed abundantly. They do not want a feeling of limitation. This is what they fear vegetarianism will cause.

We need to experience in vegetarianism a sense of completeness in the moment. Otherwise, the insecurities meat eaters bring to the relationship, because they are blocked, interact with the insecurities we bring to the relationship because we aren't blocked.

I invited vegetarians to send me their survival tips. So many of them emphasized this dilemma: how to have a feeling of abundance in food in the midst of meat eating. We *will* experience scarcity of food choices in the midst of meat eaters, but there is something we can do about it: *Be prepared.*

Being prepared is a way of saying to yourself: "I am going to experience scarcity. But I need abundance. Meat eaters cannot ensure that my needs are met. Only I can ensure that I have abundance—and that's okay."

Preparation involves positive energy—planning ahead, anticipating what will happen, knowing how to take care of your needs. Preparation energy that affirms abundance is easier to integrate into our lives than the feelings of scarcity that a meat-eating world often causes.

Survival Tips—Being Prepared

- Think ahead.
- Learn to have quick meals.
- A packed lunch is your friend.
- Be flexible. Eat whatever is okay, even if it's not a whole meal or a balanced meal. You will do better at the next meal.
- Eat plenty of fruit.
- Eat things you love.
- Offer to bring a dish.
- Make plenty of food beforehand and freeze it.
- Try to buy the cheapest things from the bulk section and treat yourself to good products and prepared foods like vegan ice cream.
- BYOF (Bring Your Own Food).
- Think pasta.
- Share recipes.

These survival tips emphasize not only being prepared, but expanding your food repertoire so that you experience the abundance a plant-based diet offers.

Survival Tips—Ensuring Abundance

- Experiment with many recipes to find the ones you really like.
- Experiment with lots of new vegetables and different spices.

- Make your diet as exciting and nutritious as possible. Eat a wide variety of foods.
- Make a real effort to find new kinds of food to eat.
- Bring a dessert. That way, you don't miss out on the fun time.

Something revolutionary exists in these tips: we must take care of ourselves—after all, it is our journey. When you take care of yourself, you reveal that you are happy—happier with this "limitation" (from the meat eater's perspective) on your diet than when you had a multitude of choices. Because, of course, you still do.

Taking Care of Ourselves

The traditional vegetarian question is "Will there be food for me?" The real question is "Do I understand how to take care of myself?" Our needs may be invisible to others, but they must not be invisible to ourselves. Self-care affirms: "I have needs. No one else can meet them. It is appropriate and necessary for me to meet them."

If you have never felt abundance in your life, if you have felt discontented and unhappy, now is the time to cherish yourself.

Survival Tips for Self-Care

- Don't be afraid to ask for ingredients lists.
- Take vitamins.
- Exercise.
- Join the local gym or start a yoga practice.
- Know the supermarket inside out.
- Follow your heart.
- Try to make eating a simple chore.
- Ask what is being served beforehand.
- Mention to people that gelatin, lard, and anchovies are animal products.

- Learn to read labels.
- Be creative!
- Use the Web for recipes and support.

You are more likely to be at peace in mixed company if you are taking care of your own needs. Your choice is happiness or martyrdom.

The Problems with Martyrdom: Accepting Scarcity

When you are not able to ensure that others will meet your needs and if you fail to be prepared to take care of your own needs, you experience martyrdom. What do I mean by martyrdom? Sacrificing your own well-being to your vegetarianism. Not being prepared. It is not spiritually nourishing for you or for others in your company. Martyrdom makes everyone unhappy. The starkest example of this was told to me by a young college student. Every year she went to her grandmother's for Thanksgiving dinner. But because everything was cooked with butter, there was absolutely nothing for her to eat but a toasted, unbuttered bagel. What did this tell everyone else, as they enjoyed their traditional, abundant meal? Her choice was scarcity. She felt left out, neglected, or martyred. The others were convinced of the impracticality, the downright unpleasantness, of following an ethical diet. I encouraged her to take care of herself by planning ahead. She should prepare something to bring, to help others see how exciting vegetarianism can be. The bagel solution is really no solution. It only confirms meat eaters' fears about vegetarianism.

If martyrdom makes you feel superior, your friends and family will notice it and feel hostile toward you. If martyrdom makes you feel alienated, your friends and family may not notice it and you will feel hostile toward them. In either case, martyrdom teaches meat eaters their fears are accurate—there is nothing that vegetarians can eat. They will believe we don't celebrate Thanksgiving because we can't.

Martyrdom may mean that you are eating poorly, which not only raises food dramas for you, but is also not healthy. You lack a balanced diet. Martyrdom is a mini-death. Should a diet that embraces "life" cause mini-deaths? Martyrdom accepts the meat eater's scarcity model as the only legitimate one. What do we do when we realize this? Overturn the scarcity model; abundance is not something I achieve by eating, but by the attitude I bring to eating: "I am glad I am a vegan, but this means that I am the one who is responsible for ensuring that my needs in this area are met. I must bring some food." This acceptance, which often feels like a step backward, and may even be tinged with grief ("No one cares enough for me to watch out for my interests"), actually becomes a step toward liberation. When you lower your expectations about food in mixed company, you have the freedom that comes with lowered expectations—you are less likely to be disappointed.

We all need a sense of abundance: a sense that we have everything we need, now, at this very moment; a sense that arises not from the quantity that is before us—whether specifically the quantity of food at a meal or in general assessing our circumstances through some quantitative measurement—but from the *quality* of inner joyfulness at being who we are this very moment. If, instead, we seem to be willing to live with scarcity, that makes us strangers. Who would choose that? We are then judged for choosing scarcity: our "constricted diet" has constricted our spirit. When we choose martyrdom, in at least this way—and perhaps in other ways, too—we accept estrangement. We become strangers.

THE STRANGER

In classic movies, the stranger's arrival in town is noticed immediately. "How'd you come to this ol' town, pardner?" The question is posed as the stranger ambles into the town's saloon. The stranger has a secret— a mission, a plan—harmful or good. He (usually a he) is just passing through, inadvertently discovers something, and triggers a chain of circumstances, or he has come looking for something, finds it, and this triggers unexpected and revelatory events. His purpose will soon come into conflict with the town. The town's residents will learn something about themselves from the conflict. Are they the loving people they thought they were? Maybe not. Did the arrival of the stranger touch off a response that is evil, revealing to themselves their own inner struggles and what they have denied? In most cases, yes.

We're strangers to meat eaters because we have changed. We have done something that they haven't. We let go of our attachment to meat as food. They don't understand, or they understand but fear stops them; they understand but can't change. No one else can know your unique process of becoming a vegetarian. In any case, a person discomforted by your vegetarianism can't relate to the process. They see the product— the vegetarianism—and it is alien. They fear the process because it is different.

Often our reasons for eliminating meat are very intense ones. We may seem like strangers because of the sheer intensity with which we answer the question "Why did you become a vegetarian?" Meat eaters often do not feel this intensity around the same issues. So a question arises: Why intensity for this and not for something else? For instance, why are you this intense about dead animals and not about the homeless or the starving?

Change is threatening. This is why strangers are not trusted when they first appear in a town. And when you become a vegetarian, people in your immediate surroundings do not welcome your change. It requires that they also have to change—change by adapting to you, the vegetarian. Your family, friends, co-workers may be secretly or overtly furious when you change, if your change is seen as saying no to a part of themselves. They also assume that anything that changes a part of the world will also change *their* part of the world. Such a change is unwelcome. The result? A slew of small, medium, and large negative encounters between you and them. These negative experiences may rebound on us—causing us to be negative in our outlook on life and in relating with others.

Negativity can be something we bring to an interaction or experience, a preexisting bitterness, suspicion, alienation. Or, it can be the outcome of an interaction. Negativity often requires two for it to gain its strength. Someone feeling negative about our decision can pull us into that vortex of unresolved emotion. We need to learn to understand ourselves when we are thrown against this negativity. Yes, there will be disappointment, frustration, rage, disillusionment, disenchantment. And we must learn to identify when we are feeling them and what to do about them. They are barometers of a situation, but they don't have to turn into a storm themselves. There can also be revelation, surprise, mystery. That is because we don't do this to *become* someone, but to *be* someone. We don't do this *against* but *for*. We don't do this only for the future, but for right now.

Survival Tips—When You Are the Stranger

- Approach meat eaters carefully.
- Try not to get angry.
- You have to have a thick skin. To most people, we are still freaks.
- Remain in control. Don't become irrational.
- Educate yourself.
- Don't try to convert others.
- Don't let anyone put you down.
- Use humor but not sarcasm.
- You don't have to explain yourself to anyone.
- Be relaxed.
- Be patient with people.
- Make your choice interesting rather than pushy.
- Stay cool.
- Be positive.
- Affirm and nurture goodness, instill others with self-love and respect.
- Love the process.

A stranger threatens the status quo. She or he sees immediately what the town has tried to deny—the corrupt sheriff, the bribe-taking mayor, the murderous banker. The stranger often exposes injustice. That's us: with our hands on our holsters, we challenge everyone we encounter. "Whoa, there, pardner," we say. "What kind of burger are you eating there?" Maybe we don't actually say it; we simply imply it with our vegetarianism. We enter the saloon and suddenly everyone realizes the saloon food is tainted. "Oh, by the way," we yell, as we jump onto our trusty steed, "I know what's going on down at the town's edge—that killing. You thought you could cover it up? Not while I'm here."

Maybe we turn on one of the townspeople and, attacking them, say, "And *who* do you think you are?" We let loose with a series of cuss words. Indeed, when it comes to vegetarians, we are often strangers because of our anger.

Anger announces; it tells us something has happened we need to pay attention to. Often anger proclaims that something is not right. Become aware of your anger. We have a right to our feelings. The first question is, What are you angry about?

Is anger a sign of powerlessness or an attempt to be powerful, judging, controlling?

Are you powerless in an eating situation, experiencing your own forced martyrdom? There's no food for you, no one notices, and everyone else is eating their food, oblivious of your needs? The question is not "Should I be feeling this anger?" You are. It is not a feeling to be denied or deemed appropriate or inappropriate; it is there—it is announcing something. The questions should be:

How can I learn more about this anger?
Can I identify the feeling and acknowledge the feeling to
    myself?
Do I need to express my anger?
Is there a way to express my anger without alienating the meat
    eaters with whom I must continue living or working?

Can I explain my anger without attacking others?

What can I do instead, if my expression of anger is not possible?

In other areas of activism, passion and outrage may be welcome. They prod, they jog, they transform. But here, something else happens. Passion and outrage lose people. Anger makes others defensive. We need to develop internal resources to handle our feelings. And this is why the question is "Are you at peace with your diet?" If we are not at peace, we confirm meat eaters' fears. Recall the fears that keep meat eaters from starting their journey. Consider them in the light of your experience:

Did you experience a separation, a break in your relationship with friends and family, a disruption of your family or inner circle? Do you feel alienation from them? Frustration, anger, disappointment? Does this meat eater with whom you are interacting trigger these feelings of alienation?

Do you experience being judged for being different? What does this make you feel?

Do you experience vegetarianism as calling attention to yourself? What transpires? What do you do?

Did you experience the unknown in becoming vegetarian?

Are you a "neophobe"? Is this keeping you from embracing the joy of vegetarianism completely? Have you settled only for converted-meat meals and familiar foods?

Have you found that your appetite is not satisfied?

Did your health improve, remain the same, or get worse?

Did you have negative experiences around the loss of security and enjoyment and identity of being a meat eater?

Did you lose the feeling of comfort, the comforts associated with eating meat, including a sense of being taken care of, of being a "child" in relationship to a parent?

Did you end up judging yourself and/or your parents?

Did you realize that your culture and your parents betrayed you?
Did you lose power and control associated symbolically with
eating meat?

If so, you are probably feeling estrangement from others and from
yourself. This estrangement will confirm to meat eaters that their fears
are legitimate.

The final set of survival tips from vegetarians exists because vegetarians know that we are susceptible to estrangement:

- Get involved. Find other people like you. Join a vegetarian
  society and really get involved with it.
- Avoid dining out with your friends when you are first converting.
- Keep your chin up.
- Don't let anyone coerce you into eating something you
  don't feel good about eating.
- Don't get down because it seems like nobody agrees with
  you. Keep in mind how much good you are doing.
- Tell your friends that it is important to you to be a vegetar-
  ian and ask that they help you.
- Know that, even if you are the only one, you are doing the
  right thing.
- Call on your vegetarian friends who understand. If you
  don't have any, find ways to meet other vegetarians.
- Write a letter to the editor.
- Live with lowered expectations. Cultivate resilience. Bounce
  back.

After all, the pertinent question is not "Are you at peace with
everyone else's diet?" The issue is only "Are you at peace with your
own diet?"

IT'S IN YOUR OWN HANDS

You did change. But, hopefully, you did not become a stranger— *that* vegetarian. You became someone who knows how to change and who can help others begin their own journeys.

Being at peace involves acting with the assurance "I can take care of myself." Not only that, but "I am comfortable with this choice. You do not have to take care of me, or worry about my food choice. In fact, let me share this wonderful food with you." Being at peace is being matter-of-fact. Being at peace lowers your expectations of others while raising your expectations for yourself. You come to view everyone as a potential vegetarian and simply get out of the way of their process of recognizing this.

Rather than feeling that we have to show, to demonstrate, to vindicate, we say, "Here I am, come to me." In this case, less is more.

The more we are at peace with our diet, the more we free others to embrace it. When I stopped talking about vegetarianism and started preparing marvelous meals, when I simply lived my life as a vegan, carrying my sourdough culture and misos with me when I went on extended visits to family, when I assumed I had to meet my own needs, and that was okay, when I created foods from that place, simply wanting to share my joy at being a vegan, it created an openness. I felt abundant, and others around me could feel it, too.

A story is told of some willful young people. One of them intensely disliked an elderly man, whom everyone else judged to be very wise. "We'll show him," the young person said. And grabbing a small bird within his two hands, he accosted the old man.

"Old man!" he called brusquely.

The old man approached him.

"Tell me, old man, is the bird in my hand living or dead?" The young man had decided that if the old man said the bird was alive, he would crush the bird in his hands and reveal that he held a dead bird. If the old man said the bird was dead, the young man would release the living bird into the air. Either way, the young man would show that the old man was wrong.

The old man appraised the young one as he stood before him. He could see the tension in the young man's arms, the hands cupped together. He watched as the young man defiantly repeated the question, "Is the bird in my hand living or dead?" The old man paused a moment and then replied:

"It's in your hands."

Will the animal live or die?

Our journey to vegetarianism has been made; now it's in their hands.

3

Repairing the Hole in Our Conscience

"Thanksgiving with a Conscience"
—TITLE OF COVER STORY ON A VEGETARIAN THANKSGIVING
IN THE *New York Times Magazine*

I f a vegetarian Thanksgiving is a Thanksgiving with a conscience, what then is a *non*vegetarian Thanksgiving? The following story provides an answer.

Traveling on an airplane once, I was seated next to a child psychologist. We had already engaged in a long, relaxed conversation about his profession and his work with troubled, gifted children. We had discussed my elementary school–age children. Then mealtime arrived. His meal of dead chicken arrived first and he began to eat it. When my vegan meal was delivered to my seat, not surprisingly, it prompted a discussion. He admitted knowing that meat eating was unethical, but still persisted in his ways. Because we had already explored some of my parenting concerns, I felt comfortable turning to him and asking what this felt like:

"What happens, then, when you sit down to eat meat?"

"I have a hole in my conscience," he said.

I thought about that, a compelling and honest answer. But I was troubled. "But our whole culture says it's okay," I responded.

"Well, we've got a collective hole in our conscience."

His statement reminded me of Erik Erikson's comment on Gandhi's vegetarianism. In his biography of Gandhi, Erikson begins by acknowledging that "the eating of animal flesh" is "an easy matter of course for most people." *Yet,* Erikson says, turning from thoughts about Gandhi to thoughts about our culture, this may not be a good thing. The eating of animal flesh, he proposes, "may yet turn out to be a problem of psycho-social evolution." Erikson believes that awareness of this problem—awareness that we have a hole in our conscience—will occur "when humankind comes to review the inner and outer consequences of having assumed the life of an armed hunter, and all the practical and emotional dead ends into which this has led us."

Wow, that's a mouthful. In fact, he says all this in one long sentence, filled with clause after clause. It is as though the structure of the sentence demonstrates how he was following his awareness about this issue. Each clause, it seemed to me when I first encountered the sentence, was Erikson's consciousness encountering the hole in his—and his culture's—conscience. We see how awareness unfolds, thought by thought, clause by clause. He acknowledges that this hole has repercussions for us individually and collectively, having both inner and outer consequences. These include "practical and emotional dead ends."

The epigraph to this book, Mary Midgley's quote about the gestalt shift, observes that meat eaters and vegetarians look at the same thing differently. We see death; they see life. Erikson, as though adding a commentary to Midgley, suggests that we are correct to see not just death, but dead ends.

What do you do when you become aware that you have a hole in your conscience? Where does this awareness go? Either you follow the awareness and become a vegetarian or try to ignore the hole and become a blocked vegetarian. Awareness interrupted is a dead end, as surely as Erikson's sentence finally came to a full stop with a period.

AWARENESS

How do we repair the hole in the conscience? The process cannot be one of simply filling the hole with information, as though we could shovel dirt to fill a hole. Consciences are not formed like this. I imagine the hole in the conscience to be like the hole in a finely knit cotton sweater. Repairing it requires adding some new thread, and interlacing it with the old. It is a delicate process. We have to start with what is there. The same is true with a meat-eating culture and individual meat eaters. We have to start with what is there. What is there is awareness. Awareness may be blocked, but it is there.

When we became vegetarians, we began to repair the hole in our conscience about animals, our bodies, and the environment. Meat eaters, in asking, "Why are you a vegetarian?" may be actually asking, "How did awareness work this change?" When we understand how the process of awareness works in us, it helps us understand why someone becomes blocked.

The movement in thought is important to recognize, and it can actually be followed in the same way that Erikson piled up clause after clause. First, something happens—a personal experience of reading, talking, seeing something, feeling something, a hint of discomfort, a spark of insight that we have a hole within us. Something makes us aware that we are eating not just "food," we are eating "meat" or dairy products. This initial thought may be momentary: "I am eating a dead cow." Or, "Why am I eating this fish?" Or, "Veal calves are the by-products of the dairy industry." Or, "I know this can't be good for my body." This is awareness.

Awareness can easily be dismissed—"I don't want to think about it at this time"—and you move your awareness elsewhere. Or you accept the insight as a gift and think, "What am I going to do with the awareness? I need to look into vegetarianism. Then I'd be [whatever spark brought awareness]: healthier/not contributing to the suffering of animals/not eating dead animals/not using up energy/grain." Awareness leads to attention.

You can feel awareness become attention. Awareness is the path your thoughts wish to take. Attention is when you let your thoughts follow their own path and you can respond to the insight they raise within without fear, rejection, or control. Let's look a little closer at an example. "Dairy. Oh, it comes from cows. Cows suffer. But I want a cheese pizza." The cheese pizza is more important and immediate than the awareness. So, I have to banish the idea of what happens to cows. But I look at the pizza and now it looks bloody. Still the desire remains. "I want the pizza. I will eat that pizza anyway! I want this pleasure now!" Afterward the thought arises: "Why did I eat that pizza? I could have had something else. Now I feel guilty. I didn't have to eat that pizza." But being blocked, I might on the following Friday go through the same cycle again. I have a closed energy circuit: I want the pizza. Therefore, I will eat the pizza and ignore my thoughts about health, animals, or the environment.

When awareness moves into attention, we have an open energy circuit. "I want the pizza. But if I eat the pizza, I am compromising my own commitment to animals [or health or the environment]. How can I keep this commitment? I could have a noncheese pizza, or I have been thinking about making pizza. What could I use as a topping?" I follow my thoughts and discover they are taking me to another place. There is no dead end. When awareness becomes attention, there is growth and flexibility, not frozenness and a sense of being caught.

Awareness interrupted, deflected, denied, becomes guilt, defensiveness, a dead end. Awareness that is followed becomes attention. Though it is thought that becoming a vegetarian requires energy, in fact, *not* becoming a vegetarian requires energy, too. The difference is that the vegetarian can follow the energy that awareness about meat eating releases, whereas the meat eater must block or redirect the energy.

After following awareness, we may feel pain, alarm, upsetness. This is what awareness can do; it opens us to the suffering of ourselves and others. Meat eaters, not being able to follow awareness, feel numb. They must deaden (dead-end) the part of them that would respond to this awareness.

It could be said that following awareness lets "flow" happen. Inner flow is a release of energy, allowing energy to follow its path. It is the liberation of energy, the opening up of channels of energy, an internal pull that we develop the ability to heed. Three characteristics can be observed in following the flow: openness, receptivity, freedom. Flow is freedom from attachments to meat eating, to old expectations; freedom from old needs. Then we can begin to repair the hole in our conscience.

But what of those individuals blocking awareness? They, too, sensed something about meat or dairy, but then diverted the energy. Yet at some level, the message comes through that their actions are inconsistent with their conscience.

If one knows one is being inconsistent, the response may be to defend oneself against this knowledge, rather than to acknowledge that one is being inconsistent. The hole gets bigger. The nonvegetarian may not be aware consciously of what she or he is doing in dancing around this hole in their conscience. "What I am doing cannot survive close scrutiny, it does not accord with my idea of my own—and others'—humanity. It clashes with the values I believe I have. So, I am going to distort this action, split it apart from everything else, and do everything to defend myself against the realization." The more people are uncomfortable with what they are doing, the more they will have to defend it.

Meat eaters must actively repress a considerable amount of information to continue eating meat. To keep that resistance operating requires quite a bit of emotional energy. They must continuously control what they have repressed so that it does not come to consciousness. To someone who is actively repressing information, a vegetarian is implicitly perceived as a threat. Our vegetarianism exposes people's repressed feelings and thoughts, and this makes them uncomfortable. We demonstrate that awareness does not have to be blocked. Holes in the conscience can be repaired.

We cannot halt a meat eater's reaction to a vegetarian, since merely announcing our vegetarianism provokes it. *You* are to blame for their awareness of discomforting feelings. You aren't telling them something new, but this is the problem. You are a reminder of something that has been postponed, justified, banished, and repressed. The interaction then becomes a battle of control, and they attempt to rid themselves of those unpleasant emotions that arise with the reminder that one does not need to eat meat. Often you, the vegetarian, the person who has reminded them of this feeling of discomfort, seem to be the *cause* of the discomfort. Once there is an external cause for this feeling, there can be an external remedy. You are the problem. If you are the problem, than meat eating isn't the problem.

This results in Erikson's inner and outer consequences of accepting being an armed hunter. Control must be maintained to keep energy from following its path.

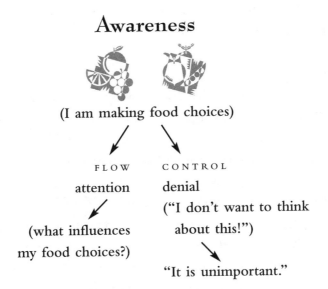

Awareness

(I am making food choices)

FLOW   CONTROL

attention   denial

(what influences   ("I don't want to think
my food choices?)   about this!")

"It is unimportant."

FIGURE 1. FLOW AND CONTROL CHART.

Denial short-circuits awareness and in its place defensiveness erupts.

Flow and control are the opposite of each other. The problem is that control has a hook—it's easier, simpler, more "real," more tangible. It's got history on its side. The payoff for staying connected to control is more immediate, but so are the frustrations.

Flow	Control
grace	blockage
faith	worry
inner	outer
no fear of failure	anxiety
process	product
life	standing still
movement from the center	movement from the past

How do meat eaters exercise control over this rebel awareness that wishes to overthrow it? By saying, "I don't want to know."

They don't want to know because then they are aware; being aware, they would have to assess how they feel; feeling the feelings (about their health, environment, or animals), they would learn how to respond to them; in responding to them, they would find they could change. In saying, "I don't want to know," each meat eater says, "Don't come between me and my self-deceptions. I want to see myself as a good person. I perceive that you have made a sacrifice for moral reasons. You threaten my sense of being a good person because I have not acted in a similar way." It does not matter that vegetarianism does not feel like a sacrifice to you. It appears that way to them.

When they interact with a vegetarian, in this way, they suggest a knowledge about themselves that they don't want to have. But they sense that we know it immediately, and if they are sensitive, they know it through our knowing. Our knowing enables them to grasp it, too. This is the crux of the problem. Through our knowing, they may see they are not doing what they tell themselves they are doing (eating humanely, eating healthily, protecting the environment). This is troubling. We reveal to them one aspect of who they are.

In response, we may be told: "How trivial, how unimportant. All this is about animals? Or the environment? Your health?" On the other hand, they may say, "Don't tell me about this, it's too upsetting." Well, it can't be both. If it is trivial, it is not upsetting. And if it is upsetting, it can't be trivial. Answer: They have made it seem trivial because it is upsetting.

People say, "Don't tell me" or "I don't want to know" because if they engaged with the knowledge, they would have to do something about it themselves. Unlike other social problems where you can praise the activists, write checks to vital groups, and support issues without other, more personal involvement, the issue of vegetarianism requires the individual's active engagement—and change.

*"I have your book, but I am afraid if I read it,
I might not be able to eat meat afterward."*

or

"I don't want to know because I would have to change."

or

*"I don't want to know because if I know, I will feel,
and those feelings make me uncomfortable."*

Nonvegetarians achieve a delicate stasis in their deflection of awareness. And so they remain blocked, and resolve to stay blocked. . . . Until they encounter a vegetarian. Then their delicate stasis is threatened.

VEGETARIANS PROMPT AWARENESS IN MEAT EATERS

It Is Mostly Unwelcome

Eating meat is generally experienced as a relationship between an individual and his or her food choices. Vegetarians know—and remind others—that there is a third, hidden dimension; namely, everything that is involved in meat production: consumption by the animals of food resources, antibiotics, etc.; environmental issues; the animals' experience and death; the people who have to work in slaughterhouses; health issues; and so on. Our presence often reminds meat eaters that something is hidden and it is not just the hidden dimension of meat production. Something is hidden within them—their awareness.

The problem of meat eating quickly becomes a problem with meat eaters. One of the major dramas of meat eating in our time is one's individual responsibility for animals' deaths, for the existence of factory farms, and for animals' suffering. Meat cannot exist without these. But meat eaters like to think they are doing what vegans are doing—eating humanely and healthily—without actually doing what vegans are doing—not eating meat or dairy. They can only believe, however, that they are eating humanely and healthily as long as there is no vegetarian around. A vegetarian in the midst of meat eaters implicitly announces, "What you claim is not what you're doing." We remind them of the hole in their conscience. Deeper than our need to eat meat is our belief in our own humanity and kindness. But the conscience is saying that there is a conflict between these two desires—to "do good"/be humane and to eat meat.

Vegetarians become reminders of what meat eaters have failed to do. Meat eaters' unresolved issues with their own meat eating encumbers their relationships. Meat eaters are not necessarily aware that this is what is happening. The world is structured to help them forget. There is a collective hole, too. Because of the collective hole, meat eating is not perceived as one of two choices: meat eating or vegetarianism. Since it is not seen as one of two choices, meat eaters rarely have to define themselves as meat eaters or acknowledge that they make a choice in their diet. The result is that the meat eating is unmarked. A meat eater usually does not see himself or herself as a meat eater until a vegetarian makes an appearance.

A vegetarian, simply by being a vegetarian, makes others aware of food choices. When you, a "vegetarian," appear, they suddenly become meat eaters. The moment they get their identity as "meat eater," it is threatened, by your vegetarianism. Take away that identity, take away their food, and what would they have? Yet you show that it can be done. This is the power of vegetarianism: something taken for granted just the way it is becomes marked, a choice.

It is our vegetarianism that is seen as separating us from them, not their meat eating. We are experienced as creating a dualism. Where once there were simply people who went out to eat, now there are different types of people who are going out to eat—vegetarians and meat eaters.

Anything that labels us and separates us into opposing groups reinforces a them/us approach, and drives a wedge into the interaction. Where there was unity in eating, there are now two sides, meat eater and vegetarian. You are seen as the cause of this and of the awareness, too. You have created the schism. Difference creates anxiety.

It may feel as though we have created this sense of divisiveness and difference. We haven't. We have caused it to come to consciousness.

It does not matter what you believe about your vegetarian or low-fat diet. It does not matter what the motivation is that brought you to this diet. The dualism between meat eater and vegetarian exists separately from you as an individual. You are on one side of the dualism and the meat eater is on the other. You set off a chain of reactions because you remind the meat eater that there is a choice.

In announcing that you are a vegetarian, you are saying, "I'm not blocked in this area anymore." And de facto you are saying, "You still are." Besides all the energy they are using to block *their* own vegetarianism, they are expected to be receptive to your *unblocked* vegetarianism. For many, this feels impossible.

ENCOUNTERING BLOCKED VEGETARIANS

While it might be tempting to spend time asking, "Why aren't you here?" it is more profitable to figure out, "Why are they there?" The answer is that something is keeping them blocked.

Why Meat Eaters Stay Blocked

- Taste: Many people enjoy the taste of cooked flesh.
- Change takes *too much* energy: "I don't have the time or the energy. Cooking is a chore. Meat is simple to cook. You have to work so much harder for a vegetarian meal."
- Ignorance: "I don't know how to begin."
- It's trivial: "I don't think it's necessary" or "We're talking about animals here! Cows and chickens and pigs! Who cares what happens to them?"
- Passivity: "I have a sense that I don't have the ability to change." This is reinforced by the general passivity of American culture. We have become a community of "watchers." A passive public who follow the storyline, whether it be O. J., Princess Diana, or President Clinton. We need villains and victims but don't want to be either. We want to be voyeurs, not the actors.
- Laziness: "It's too hard to do this. And it would be too inconvenient if I did."
- Whether age 25, 35, 45, 55, 65, or 75: "I'm too old to change."
- A sense of fragility: "I cannot handle anything else! I can't handle any more changes!" Some people have been so damaged that they decide "an animal's suffering is not comparable to mine. I cannot care about what is happening to them. I can only handle what is happening to me." Or they think, "I have changed so much of myself already, I just can't change anything else."
- It is too difficult, requiring too much mental work: "I don't want to put myself through a new way of thinking."
- Food issues: "I'll feel cheated if deprived of any kinds of food. I love to have free food. I cannot bear to give up any choice."
- Comfort: "I am comfortable this way."

- Cost: "It's too expensive."
- Apathy: "I don't care about what is happening to the animals used for food. I don't care about what it does to my body."
- Denial: "I don't want to admit that I was lied to and that I am lying to myself."
- A sense of meaninglessness about an individual's behavior: "What's the use? My changing won't have any effect. The animals are going to die anyway."
- Apocalyptical thinking: "I'm going to die anyway" (or "The planet is going to die"), so "I might as well enjoy myself."
- Someone else can't change: "I'd become a vegetarian, but my husband needs meat."
- A need for the status quo: "I know who I am. If I change, I won't know who I am."
- Priorities: "We have to help humans first!"

All of these reasons remind us that it is easier to *be* someone than to *become* someone else.

Yet there you stand: *you* became someone else. You stopped eating meat. How did you repair the hole when they can't? The nonvegetarian will have to explain your changing somehow without its reflecting on themselves.

HOW MEAT EATERS EXPLAIN YOUR DIET

Vegetarianism is only one part of who we are. This part becomes magnified in vegetarian–meat eater relationships. The question meat eaters struggle with is how this part relates to the rest of who you are. Inevitably, they come up with an explanation. It may not be accurate, but it is comforting to them, because it confirms them in their blocked status.

If you want to learn what a meat eater thinks about you, it will be revealed in their explanation. In explaining why we changed, their assumption often is that vegetarianism expresses a negative aspect of one's personality rather than a positive one. It is something to analyze and resist rather than accept. This is a way to deflect attention from their own practices of meat eating, but it also may reveal the thorny, prickly areas of our own personalities. After all, our personalities affect how we respond to giving up meat. We may respond tenaciously, laconically, bitterly, enthusiastically, evangelically. You may be embittered, impatient, and also a vegetarian. You may be accepting, nonjudgmental, and a vegetarian. To explain your vegetarianism, these aspects of your personality may become a focus, a redirection of the vegetarian impulse into a more controllable area—not who you have become but who you have always been. They don't see vegetarianism as transformative, but as something that unleashes your old, predictable demons. If you are fastidious in life, you are "fussy" in eating. It has to do specifically with who you are, not with the legitimacy of the diet regardless of the individual. These explanations can be merciless. They explain your vegetarianism in such a way that vegetarianism is bracketed by inescapable facts of your personality.

Nonvegetarians usually explain your vegetarianism by mixing three things together: trying to defend what is blocking them, attacking your personality tics, and labeling you—pigeonholing you into one of several "types" of vegetarians. They resort to this because it makes the "you" you have become more understandable. A label is interposed between who you really are and how your vegetarianism is experienced. The label is a buffer. If you are seen as having a legitimate concern about meat eating, you will be experienced as saying something to them, something they do not want to hear. Stereotypes are so much easier on their conscience. They begin with whatever group we are associated with, whether by birth or choice: so it may be thought "it's a woman thing" or a teenage girl thing. If he's a man, well, he's gay. If she's a person of color, "it's her 'tradition'"; if he's white, "he doesn't have to worry about his tradition." If the person is rich, "she can afford to be a vegetarian." If the person is poor, "he doesn't have a choice." Besides the obvious social groups to which we gravitate, explanations of vegetarianism also classify us into different types.

MEAT EATERS' CLASSIFICATION OF VEGETARIANS

The Ascetic

An ascetic, according to *The American Heritage Dictionary of the English Language,* "renounces material comfort and leads a life of austere self-discipline." An ascetic is admired for holding to her principles, but the life she has decided to live is too hard for any average Jane or Joe to aspire to. Several things happen when a vegetarian is considered an ascetic:

1. You are admired, but it is believed that what you have done cannot be achieved by anyone else.
2. The belief takes hold that to be vegetarian requires giving up the enjoyment of all foods that are pleasurable (meat eating = pleasure).
3. Then it is assumed that the vegetarian expects you to do the same, which leads to the perception of another type: the Puritan.

The Puritan

This is almost a subset of ascetic, but constitutes its own type because the Puritan does not arouse positive feelings. They fear that you want to deprive them of their enjoyment. Your reasons are not seen as admirable. Your self-denial is explained in this way: "She doesn't enjoy anything, and she doesn't want anyone else to either." One reason vegetarians are thought to be against pleasure is because they have the potential to destroy the pleasures of the meal for a meat eater. This potential exists precisely because meat eaters are blocked. They don't know the pleasures of *our* meals, but they do know the pleasure we have deprived them of. They now cannot eat their own meat without awareness of our not doing so.

The Puritan is perceived as humorless and as deriving no enjoyment from living. Because of this, the Puritan is always suspected of wanting to deny others their pleasure. In the face of the assumption that it is our right to maximize our pleasure, the Puritan is seen as legislating and controlling.

The Bambi Vegetarian

As individuals, we grow up learning to deny the legitimacy of our feelings. Being matter-of-fact about animals' deaths is a sign of health and maturity in our culture. Thus vegetarianism is thought to be a problem of misplaced or immature emotions. The implication is that responding to suffering is out of place.

It is assumed you're just too sensitive; you never got over those Disney movies of your childhood. You don't accept loss. You don't know how to focus your emotions properly on "real" problems. In fact, you are just too emotional. You're told: "Come on! You care about cows and pigs? Get real." Animal-loving is seen as a sign of arrested development. "Grow up."

A subset of the Bambi vegetarian that exploits gender issues is the "wimp" or "fruit." This type is male and his sexuality (presumed to be heterosexual) and maleness are seen as being undercut by his vegetarianism, which is attributed to his being a "feeling type" rather than a macho man (who is not supposed to exhibit feelings). If the man is gay, meat eaters may assume that vegetarianism is one aspect of his gayness, rather than understanding that a man who has worked out his sexual identity has gained experience in working on identity issues, of which vegetarianism is one.

The "Freak"

You eat strange. You have weird beliefs. You like tofu, for heaven's sake. You separate yourself from everyone else. You alienate meat eaters, so you must be alienated. "I could never do it. I don't want to do it, and

I don't know how you can do it." A derivative type, the "Birkenstock" vegetarian or "California" vegetarian: You're still living in the '60s, eating granola and raw foods. Your choices are incomprehensible, thus the label. "What else is there to give up?" "You actually like this stuff?"

The Holier-Than-Thou Vegetarian

You are angry and judgmental, holier-than-thou and godlike in your wrathful nature. Nonvegetarians feel your anger. Your anger fills all the space between you and them. They say: "You make me feel guilty." They think: "Who are *you* to make *me* feel guilty?" They conclude, "You are a vegetarian because you see yourself as better than everyone else." The "vegan police" are a subset of the holier-than-thou vegetarian.

The Phobic Vegetarian

"You just have a hang-up about food." You are neurotic. Self-obsessed. It's a rejection of your

    sexuality
    your father
    fallen nature
    [fill in the blank]

If you are a teenage girl and thin, you are accused of becoming a vegetarian as a cover for your anorexia.

What does each of these types teach us about blocked vegetarians?

The *ascetic* and *Puritan* labels tell us that meat eaters fear their own suffering. They cannot require something difficult of themselves.

The *Bambi* label tells us that the suffering of animals in factory farms cannot be heard. Meat eaters project onto us their fear of relating to animals who are victims of meat eating. Rather than confront those concerns (which would then force them to reconsider their diet), they try to dismiss the vegetarian as sentimental, emotional, and irrational.

The *freak* label says, "You're different and I don't want to be different. I don't want to separate myself from others. I cannot understand you."

The *holier-than-thou* label, which will be expressed as "Who do you think you are?" or, less confrontationally, "You make me feel guilty," reveals that the meat eater has issues around judging him- or herself.

With the *phobic* label, much is going on. It reminds us that we live in a therapeutic age, and so there is a gravitation toward explaining all food-related concerns as psychological issues. Everything's going to be seen as an individual hang-up rather than as a political recognition and engagement. It is often assumed that the catholic eater, the generic eater, the gourmand, who is willing to try anything and so is open to new tastes, does not have issues with food. Only those who actively change their diets, and thus appear to be worried about food, seem to have issues with food. When Julia Child characterized vegans as having a hang-up with food, she captured this viewpoint. But this drive to be seen as unconcerned about food is suspiciously like protesting *too* much.

And so friends, co-workers, parents, children pathologize the decision, trying to find out "what is wrong with you." You may be feeling, "*Wrong?* Finally something feels right to me!" But for them, the untangible—awareness—has to be translated into the tangible, an explanation. Why are you different? It is much safer to attribute it to anything but awareness, since awareness can operate equally in everyone, but doesn't.

When you hear the comments associated with each type—for instance, "Grow up," you can then say, "Oh, I see, they think I am a Bambi vegetarian. That means they are uncomfortable with their feelings about animals and must not acknowledge them."

Now the catch in this analysis is that, in your interactions with meat eaters, you may indeed be manifesting aspects of one of these types unknowingly.

Have you unprocessed anger? You become holier-than-thou.

Are you oppressed by how unfriendly the world seems to a vegetarian? You may be perceived as a Puritan, or phobic. You are either legislating or hung up about food.

"EVERYONE KNOWS"

Most meat eaters, of course, will let you know how they size you up. This often occurs in a certain statement that follows a formula:

"Everyone knows you just have a hang-up about food."

This damns at the beginning and the end of the sentence. Not only do you have a problem, but you are apparently the only one who doesn't recognize it!

The formula looks like this:

A knows B about YOU!

A is *who knows.*

B is *what they know* about YOU! It is knowledge that is supposed to shame you.

This formula tells us that they are trying to figure out what's wrong with *us,* rather than *our culture.* Remember: if it is about us, it doesn't have to be about them. Thus, a frontal assault occurs:

A:

Everyone	knows you . . .
All your friends	know . . .
The whole family	knows . . .
Your co-workers	know . . .

B:

you have a hang-up with food.

you never got over the death of your bunny/chicken/horse/pig.

you are trying to control everyone's food habits.

you aren't committed to the family tradition.

you love animals but you hate people.

you are doing this to hurt your mother/grandmother/father.

you just want to be different.

you just want to be difficult.

you just want some attention.

you just want to rebel.

Etc.

Take one phrase from A and add one phrase from B. For instance: "Everyone knows you just want attention."

Here is a classic drama enacted in numerous households, workplaces, college dorms, and so on across the country. This is baiting you because it is making *you* the issue. Don't take the bait. Don't respond by saying: "I don't want attention! That's ridiculous." Or, depending on the attack: "I *don't* have a hang-up with food! What do you mean?" Or, "Of course I care about the family tradition!"

None of these responses diffuses the attack. They only intensify it. These responses accept the basic premise of the statement. Not only that: in accepting the validity of the charges that make you the target and in protesting them, you will sound emotional, upset. They will have won. "We said you had a problem, and you are showing us you have a problem. Why would you get upset if there weren't a problem? There *is* something wrong with you, that is what we are saying. . . . Wrong with *you,* and not with us. We don't have a hole in our conscience!"

What should you do instead? *Step aside.* Don't let the statement land on you. To all of these charges, you can always say: "People adopt vegetarianism for a wide range of reasons, some perhaps better than others. Undeniably, there are good reasons to be vegetarian." And leave it at that. The conversation might then take this turn: "What, is that all you are going to say?"

To which you reply, "Yes."

This is not your drama and don't let it become yours.

To the charges that "everyone knows you have a hang-up with food," or "everyone knows you never got over the death of your pony," you can simply say: "How very kind of them. I am deeply touched."

Another way to describe this formula is that nonvegetarians are explaining your vegetarianism by classifying you into a "type": "Everyone knows you are a vegetarian because you are [a description of one of the types]."

Thus, if you are seen as an ascetic vegetarian, you don't enjoy eating. If you are seen as a holier-than-thou vegetarian, you like to judge other people. If you are seen as phobic, you have a hang-up. And so on.

To any of these statement—those following either the simple A–B formula, or "Everyone knows you are 'X' type"—you have a choice of responses. You can respond by saying: "I've noticed that a lot of people, who generally are very nice and respectful, say insensitive or mean things to me about my diet. I wonder whether this may reflect their own conflicts about what is the most ethical way to eat."

Or you can say: "I've noticed that people often confuse food issues with thoughtful decisions about [health/environment/animals]. Why do you think everyone makes that mistake?"

This is a much more sophisticated turn, which does not dignify the attack with a direct answer. But it continues the conversation, which is something you might not want to do at a time when you know the other person is feeling defensive. You can deflect the implicit criticism and offer some guidance, but you need to be careful not to allow this response to pull you into a debate: "Hmmm. That's a strange observation. ["Strange" can be a very disarming response.] I've never thought of that. Perhaps it's true, but I really don't think that is a major motivation for my diet. I suspect strongly that my diet simply reflects my deep ethical convictions regarding animal treatment, environmental protection . . . [etc.]."

Or, you can choose a traditional avoidance response to defensiveness: postponement. Choose one of the other responses and postpone the confrontation. After all, the meat eaters are postponing something, too: acknowledging the hole in their conscience.

POSTPONEMENT

How comfortable to postpone consciousness and to find excuses for not acting! We ourselves may know such postponements and hesitations all too well.

Signs of a Blocked Vegetarian

"Oh, I wish I could do that, but it's just so hard."

"I've been waiting till I'm not so busy, less stressed, [etc.]."

"I thought about it once."

"I've been thinking about it myself."

"I tried it once."

"Seeing you makes me feel guilty."

Awareness that one has a hole in one's conscience and not addressing the hole prompts the discovery of painful and uncomfortable aspects about ourselves—aspects we would prefer not to know. It is painful to know that we failed to live up to our own expectations. When we feel the pain of this failure, we have two choices: either to examine the conditions that caused us to fail and determine to create the conditions for success, or to reorient our own expectations for our behavior and actions.

It may seem easier to reconcile oneself to the hole in the conscience rather than sustain awareness of what has caused this rupture. *Thus, it becomes more painful to experience the failure of will or consciousness, than to be aware of meat eating.* It is safer to believe "*I don't need to do this*" than "*I can't do it.*" So the belief evolves that no change is necessary. This belief holds true, as long as a meat eater interacts only with other meat eaters. But, upon encountering a vegetarian, the rationalization stumbles—there stands someone who hasn't postponed. What was postponed then becomes a source of either guilt or defensiveness.

In the presence of a vegetarian, meat eaters may be reminded of decisions they made at one time about vegetarianism but never accomplished. They are aware, but they have not acted. They know, but they fail to change. It is hard to learn this about oneself: "I have failed to live up to my own expectations."

Were their reasons for postponement legitimate in their eyes, now, given your presence and your ability to let go of meat? You are the reminder of what has not been done. You changed. They didn't. Their unresolved relationship to meat eating—the hole in their conscience—now encumbers your relationship.

Meat eaters postpone becoming vegetarians because they think change is hard. *Not* changing is even harder. They just haven't discovered this yet.

4

Judgment, Guilt, and Anger

My brother-in-law Merv is a minister and marriage counselor. One summer I was helping him rehabilitate an old house. A contractor arrived around 9:00 A.M. to give him an estimate on a furnace. Later—so much later that I was ready to quit for lunch—Merv reappeared. Clearly, the conversation had taken longer than he had anticipated. Explaining what had been so time-consuming, he observed, "When you tell someone you are a minister, they say, 'Let me tell you about my faith.' When you tell someone you are a marriage counselor, they say, 'Let me tell you about my marriage.'"

I added, "And when you tell someone you are a vegetarian, they say, 'I don't eat *that much* meat!'"

We both laughed.

A blocked vegetarian does not want to be reminded that she or he is blocked. In everyday interactions, such reminders may not occur. Enter a vegetarian. Now the vegetarian is the reminder that one has made a decision not to change. People generally want a self-image that tells them they are good, worthy, and moral individuals. We vegetarians threaten this self-image. The vegetarian is experienced as judging the meat eater simply because she is a vegetarian. This dynamic actually has nothing to do with the vegetarian in question but everything to do with what she represents—someone who integrated awareness with action. Our acting—becoming a vegetarian—provokes defensiveness on the part of the meat eater who has failed to act.

Meat eaters bring to their relationship with vegetarians their own unresolved guilt about continuing to eat meat. They feel they have to defend their own practices. Consider this story from a vegan in Brooklyn:

> I went to visit my parents; my brother was in the kitchen cooking. As I entered the foyer I am greeted with, "Shut up! I am eating it anyway. . . ." I was confused, so I asked, "What?" My brother launched into a rampage of excuses as to why he was going to eat veal. "You know," I responded, "it is the guilty conscience that speaks the loudest."

Or this from California:

> I have spent a lot of time talking to people about the issues at a vegetarian information table on the boardwalk at Venice Beach, California. The majority of people who come up to me are not really interested in learning about vegetarianism. It seems that most of them just want to pick a verbal fight. At times they even yell, scream, and call my partner and me names. This can be very agitating, and most of the time I just ignore them or I tell them that they would not be picking a fight with me if they were okay with their dietary beliefs. I feel that even the combative people who approach vegetarians are in search of change, although they themselves don't know it.

As we saw in the previous chapter, awareness that is followed becomes attention. Awareness interrupted, deflected, or denied transforms into negative energy. "I have a hole in my conscience that allows me to eat meat. The more I understand of the hole in my consciousness, the more compelled I am to stop eating meat. But I don't want to stop eating meat! Yet the more I understand of the hole, the more pressure there is to stop. I will resist this pressure." Blocked energy is expressed through emotions such as guilt and anger. People who say, "You make me feel guilty" or who act belligerently to you are saying, "I'm stuck."

Resisting an internal pull takes a lot of work; it is working against the flow. The old needs continue to control the individual. Three characteristics of resisting the flow are judgment, guilt, and anger. It is an internal dynamic. Suspicion arises toward someone from the outside who appears in a position to judge; someone who followed the flow. What stands between them? The blocking force.

THE BLOCKING FORCE

The primary problem for blocked vegetarians is that something is keeping them from repairing the hole in their conscience. This something is probably a combination of the reasons identified in Chapter 3 and the fears meat eaters have about vegetarianism, discussed in Chapter 2. Together these are *the blocking force*. If it remains unscrutinized, it will grow in power.

Interactions with individuals who are blocking the flow may proceed in ways akin to this:

Most of my frustrating experiences stem from one friend of mine who is a very socially conscious individual in issues of human rights. However, in terms of animal welfare, her awareness is lacking. Her attitude toward meat eating is that humans will evolve one day but right now it is "natural" to eat meat. . . . It is an argument that disguises the real issue, which is that she really likes/craves the taste of meat and does not want to give it up for more expensive/worse-tasting alternatives (though I have tried to explain to her that this is not the case). In my company she will eat meat even after we have just had a discussion on the issue and it angers me but makes me disappointed and sad also. We have often been in heated arguments over the issue and are both left frustrated.

After such interactions, one feels exhausted, disappointed, sad, outraged, frustrated. For many years I walked away from conversations feeling this. That is because I presumed that no matter how well crafted the other person's arguments were in defense of eating meat, dairy products, and eggs, I had better arguments against them. I didn't realize that these arguments were a part of their protection plan against *the blocking force*. Nothing, absolutely nothing, was coming near the real reasons for staying blocked.

If an individual senses that what blocks them is not as legitimate as they keep telling themselves it is, they will already feel defensive. But you are going to be seen as the agent of their discomfort. Defensiveness represents a quarrel with their own conscience. Defensiveness is a no-win situation for us because it protects the status quo.

It is not the *content* of the friend's defenses that is important here: it is the *dynamics*. These dynamics are actually in the meat eater's interest, because she gets to defend her ground. She doesn't want either the vegetarian or herself to get too near to her blocking force. Instead of having to examine this blocking force, she gets to use that energy toward the vegan friend. This allows her to avoid what is really needed: her own internal conversation.

Her own internal dialogue might go something like this:

Insight: "Gee, I'm eating a dead animal."

Response: "Yes, but I don't want to change. I like the taste of meat!"

Insight: "But this can't be very good for you, either. Look at all those health statistics."

Response: "I can't handle any more change. I don't want to learn anything new. I don't want to give up meat."

Insight: "Well, what are you going to do with me, then?"

Response: "Don't you get it? I don't want to change and I won't. So I am just going to ignore you. Push you down and keep you out of my thoughts."

Insight: "I'm not going to go away that easily."
Response: "We'll see about that!"

This is the blocking force at work. When it is externalized, the blocking force becomes defensiveness. This then actually protects meat eaters from their own sense of failure, of having let themselves down. When you come on the scene, now there is something they can do with their inner war. They can take it out into the world. They have someone to blame for their feelings and an arsenal of warring skills they have used against themselves. The blocking force leaps to battle.

Essentially, the vegetarian says, explicitly or implicitly, "You're eating a dead animal. It's not good for you, or the earth, or the animal." The meat eater is well equipped to handle these arguments—because there has already been an internal argument along those lines. We inadvertently fall right into line with their accustomed way of handling vegetarianism: argument, avoidance, and then suppression. They relate to us as they do to that part of themselves they refuse to interact with. In this process, we actually bolster their defenses. They get to externalize that inner argument, which releases for them the energy that they have been repressing. Like a pressure cooker releasing steam, instead of having to cook the insights through their own process, they get to release them, and we encounter their raw feelings.

They are letting you take on the role of judge/critic. This relieves them of being their own judge, listening to their own insights, and discovering that they can indeed change. This gives their blocking force greater strength. It has dug in for the duration. In suppressing inner and outer arguments, the meat eater walks away cleansed of guilt, freed of anger, and relieved.

SHOULDA . . .

Each of us—whether vegetarians or meat eaters—has an inner critic, in psychological terms a superego, filling our heads with *shoulds* and *oughts*. The superego tells us what we "shoulda" done or should be doing. It is a partly conscious, and largely unconscious, moral system. It speaks through the voice of conscience.

The superego is good and necessary. It evolves as we mature. A mature superego isn't swallowing whole the commands our society gave us. Instead, it is integrating them with our own identity, our own experience, and the knowledge we have gained as we mature.

The process of constantly integrating new information is a process of growth. A healthy superego enables us to balance the demands of self and the needs of others. We are able to experience ourselves as embedded within a fabric of life, with responsibilities and rewards. The struggle always is finding the balance between the self and others. We constantly ask ourselves, "What is it that I want to do, given my commitment to myself and also to others?"

For instance, someone becomes aware that animals suffer. He has to integrate that knowledge into his mature and complex superego. But here is information that can't be integrated—not if one wants to continue eating meat and continue to see oneself as a moral individual. A part of the individual is aware that the information has not been integrated. What "shoulda" he be doing?

Enter a vegetarian. We seem to be telling the meat eater exactly what he "shoulda" be doing: become a vegetarian. Here we are representing that which, when unintegrated, is an immense burden. This makes the meat eater feel even more embattled. Meat eaters assume we are judging them.

Interactions in which vegetarians are accused of judging meat eaters are some of the most frustrating experiences for vegetarians. A vegetarian does not necessarily come into a relationship and say, "I expect you to give up eating meat." The meat eater assumes that expectation is there. This is because meat eaters are already judging themselves. They use your vegetarianism to judge themselves. It is a process we cannot halt, since merely announcing our vegetarianism provokes it.

The vegetarian appears before a meat eater as an embodied "shoulda." "You should not be eating meat," we appear to be saying, simply by demonstrating that one can survive without meat. "You don't need meat. Why are you eating meat?" We don't have to say a word about meat eating for our presence to be a reminder of these kinds of thoughts. This dynamic is rarely liberating.

When a meat eater reacts defensively to you, it tells you something more than "I am a blocked vegetarian." It also tells you, "I am struggling with my relationship to my conscience."

Thus people delegate the role of the superego to us. They aren't really saying, "You make me feel like a bad person because I eat meat." They are saying, "You make me feel like a bad person because I am insecure about my decision to eat meat, and you seem secure in your decision not to eat it, and your security, as well as my own conscience, threatens me."

When we experience expressions of guilt or anger from someone, they are emphatically saying, "Don't remind me of this shoulda!"

SHOULDA, COULDA . . . *DIDN'T*

The progression of an unblocked vegetarian:

"I know about meat eating; I *should* become a vegetarian." (Awareness)

"I know about meat eating; I *could* become a vegetarian." (Reflection)

"I know about meat eating; I *have* become a vegetarian." (Action)

But, with a blocked vegetarian; the final statement becomes:

"I know about meat eating; I *didn't* become a vegetarian."

As one teenage friend says, "Shoulda, coulda . . . *didn't*."

Didn't ruptures the flow of consciousness. Justification emerges in its place:

"I didn't become a vegetarian because of [X] (whatever is blocking me)."

Consequently, "[X] is more important than vegetarianism."

And since [X] is more important than vegetarianism, the flow of awareness toward becoming a vegetarian must be controlled.

To most meat eaters this reasoning is sound. And as long as they are living among meat eaters, few will be challenged. But face-to-face with a vegetarian, "shoulda, coulda . . . *didn't*" seems less legitimate.

What was that reason that minimized the flow toward vegetarianism? "Because I'm so busy"? "Because life is so stressful"? By your presence, they now have to ask themselves, "Is [X] really legitimate?" Their unresolved relationship to [X] now encumbers your relationship. Not your vegetarianism, but [X], stands between you. And since it must not be spoken of, something else must become the center of attention.

Unblocked vegetarians like you reveal that whatever is [X]—no matter how strong a force in the life of an individual—can be dealt with, can come under the pull of vegetarianism and be transformed. The response of most meat eaters to having that pointed out is not "Thank you for teaching me this" but "Don't come between me and my self-deceptions!"

THE ROLE OF GUILT

Guilt can help us grow.

First, you have *awareness.* You are aware that you feel guilty.

Second, you *reflect* on this. What is causing my guilt? What is it telling me about my behavior? Should I change my behavior and/or compensate for my behavior?

Third, you *act.* You use your guilt to inform yourself, and then you align your behavior.

As a vegetarian, I was aware of the suffering of cows and chickens in their "production" of milk and eggs, and I felt guilty that I wasn't a vegan. I had to interrogate the guilt. Was it appropriate or inappropriate?

Given my knowledge of the lives of animals, the guilt was appropriate. It was telling me something that I needed to learn. Since the guilt was appropriate, what was I going to do? Change or not change? After *reflection,* was I going to *act*? At first, I did not act. I was aware of those guilty feelings. They did not go away. I got tired of feeling guilty and realized the only way to release myself from this guilt was by acting.

You can fool yourself into thinking you have progressed through these three steps when you haven't.

First, some people aren't aware of feeling guilty.

Second, some are aware, but won't reflect on it.

Third, some reflect, but won't act.

Some people use guilt to *avoid* taking any action. They think the expression of guilt is all that is necessary. This is a manipulative guilt reaction. They manipulate themselves into thinking they've done something they haven't:

I have a hole in my conscience. (Awareness)
To live a life with integrity, I need to become a vegetarian.
   (Reflection)
But I can't because of [X]. (Inaction)
So I will feel guilty because I have made [X] more important
   than vegetarianism. (A manipulative guilt reaction)

In this progression, guilt becomes a detour away from consciousness. People feel guilty instead of dealing with the feelings that prompt the guilt. Your vegetarianism says something about them: you changed, they did not—and that, too, is a choice.

I have an older friend who sometimes joins me for a meal at church. Every time she sits down with some form of meat on her plate, she turns to me and says, "I always feel so guilty when I see you." I have not said anything to her. I do not need to. I am not doing anything to catalyze that guilt except living my life. But in simply living my life I demonstrate that it can be done. She could change if she so desired. If growth is going to happen, she has to examine what causes the guilt. Is it legitimate or not? What she is saying to me, each and every time we have this interaction is, "I don't want to change, but at least I feel guilty about not changing." Feeling guilty is reassuring. It says, "I *am* moral. I *do* have sensibilities." The sensation of guilt restores her sense of herself as a moral person despite the hole in her conscience.

THE ROLE OF ANGER

Why do meat eaters get angry at vegetarians? Let's follow the internal process that may be happening:

I know I have a hole in my conscience.
I need to become a vegetarian.
But I can't because of [X].
So you think vegetarianism is more important than [X]?
How *dare* you say that *my* [X] is less important than vegetarianism!

This is a familiar experience for many vegetarians. As one young woman observed in a letter to me:

The other common experience I have is that someone will ask me to explain why I am a vegan and then hurtle off into self-righteous indignation, claiming that I am "preaching" and demanding respect for his (usually) view that meat eating is okay.

This position—"How dare you tell me that my [X] is less important than vegetarianism"—accounts for the sense that vegetarians love animals more than humans. This is because nonvegetarians feel that this unscrutinized but intimate part of themselves, this "[X]," is an essential part of them and cannot see themselves living differently from their current situation. [X] presses too strongly upon them. Yet you appear to be telling them that [X] is not as valid as they claim. They think to themselves, "What is vegetarianism anyway? It's there because of concern about harm to animals. So you care about animals more than you care about me (represented in my [X])! I knew it!"

Following closely behind this reasoning is this reaction: "How *dare* you say that *my* [X] is less important than vegetarianism! *Who* do you think you are?" When you hear that question—"Who do you think you are?"—watch out! You are dealing with a frantic blocked vegetarian.

A meat eater may associate several painful emotions with being blocked. These may include: annoyance, dejection, intimidation, tension, vulnerability, uneasiness, insecurity, skepticism, apprehension, suspicion, alarm, awe, reluctance, anxiety, impatience, nervousness, perplexity, helplessness, constriction, bewilderment, confusion, immobilization, ambivalence, awkwardness, puzzlement, hesitancy, surprise, depression, bitterness, terror, fear, guilt. Most of us are not practiced at identifying or discriminating among these various, and often painful, feelings.

In responding to discomforting feelings, we have at least four options:

1. Ignore them and hope they go away. (They don't.)
2. Get angry.
3. Identify the feelings and explore them. For instance: "I feel uncomfortable. I am feeling that way because of [X]. What is causing [X]?"
4. Identify the feeling and remind yourself that later, in a non-stressed atmosphere, you can explore them.

Unfortunately, anger short-circuits the awareness, reflection, action model available to us in steps 3 and 4. How does anger become the emotion of choice?

Feelings such as the ones I have suggested meat eaters feel have a "charge," an emotional energy. When we don't acknowledge what we are feeling, these charges floating around inside of us begin to build up. Instead of feeling uncertain and flustered, suddenly someone feels frustrated, uptight, tense. This then gets funneled into an emotion that releases the charges: anger. Often, when experiencing uncomfortable feelings, our tendency is to blame others. Finding an object, someone to blame for causing these feelings, allows the feelings to be released, and simultaneously externalizes them: The problem isn't an individual's uneasiness but someone else's vegetarianism!

We know what to do with anger. Anger can have a target outside itself. Anger gives the feeling of power; it also wards off other, more nuanced feelings. Anger replaces feelings of vulnerability with feelings of righteousness and indignation. Physically, it makes one feel strong: adrenaline flows with it; muscles contract to it. If one is feeling passive in the face of another's actions, judgments, or comments, anger enables the feeling of action and vitality. In this case, anger displaces whatever facility for introspection the nonvegetarian might have had. You are the most likely target.

Both guilt and anger reveal how the person is failing to respond to superego issues in their lives. It is in your best interest to get out of the way! Otherwise, you become the issue.

YOU BECOME THE ISSUE

Our interactions with meat eaters must presume that the process of deadening/dead-ending is at work, and not aid and abet it. We help them in the process whenever we allow them to make *us* the issue. When we are the issue, they don't have to be. Their awareness becomes interpersonal; their conflict becomes one between us; their feelings can turn toward us. The inner conflict becomes an outer conflict. It's much safer that way. The energy required to evoke change is drained off in external conflict. *We* become the problem, not awareness. We have to avoid ways that keep us as targets.

Once there is an external cause for the feelings a meat eater is feeling, the remedy also is external to them. You are the problem. If you are the problem, then being blocked is not the problem. One vegetarian complained:

> *When the conversation shifts to veganism, they automatically look at your shoes, your clothes, etc. They try to make themselves feel better by ripping apart the messenger instead of looking at themselves. And who said I was trying to convert you anyway? I thought we were just talking.*

The response of someone who feels judged is to judge another. This displaces the focus. It is reactionary. But this is what meat eaters usually bring to their relationship with us: reactionary personal politics.

As one vegetarian observed: "I have noticed that when you tell someone you are a vegetarian, they will go out of the way to insult you." This tells you that meat eaters are defending themselves against their own inner process: as long as it is about you, it is not about them. If they keep the focus on you, your thoughts, your beliefs, they don't have to examine their own thoughts. Feeling judged, they reverse the situation and try to take on the role of judging us. They search for the vegetarian's inconsistency. Thus we are peppered with questions such as:

Well, why are you wearing leather?
What about plants?
What about 35mm film?

Trying to find some inconsistency in vegetarians is a process of displacement for the blocked vegetarian. Suddenly your moral inconsistencies become much more important than theirs. You come under intense scrutiny because you've become the moral compass. There is also often a lingering distrust of anyone who is a moral compass. However, if it recurs over time, there can be an upside to this desire to find a vegetarian's inconsistency. Nonvegetarians have to pay attention to the vegetarian's lifestyle. Then, by paying attention, they begin to realize how many ways animals are oppressed. They say, "You can't eat Jell-O? Or marshmallows? Not even *Altoids*?" "What's wrong with milk?" The search for inconsistency becomes a consciousness-raising experience. What you can offer the conflicted meat eater is a sense of equanimity: This is who I am. This is what I believe. This is how a person lives who becomes aware of guilt, reflects on it, and then acts.

Most often, though, we are made the issue. Simply by being a vegetarian you remind them that they are blocked. So what's a vegetarian to do?

WHAT'S A VEGETARIAN TO DO?

It is not your role to fill the hole in someone else's conscience, only to give them the space and the tools to do so themselves. Trying to make someone responsible preempts their own responsibility. When we are self-righteous we don't offer any empty space, we are too filled. The issue is not one of *control,* that is, controlling others' decisions; this is the meat-eating model, in which a choice is never offered at the time meat eating begins. Children are not asked, "Do you want to eat a burger made of a dead cow or a veggie burger?" Our goal is not to replicate this controlling model.

Meat eaters do not have to experience *our* vegetarianism; they have to experience the way vegetarianism touches *them.* One man offers an example of how this can happen:

> *I had a friend once whom I hadn't seen in years. While we made dinner plans over the phone, I mentioned that I was a vegetarian. That evening, as I sat across from her at the dinner table, she said that she had eaten a Whopper that afternoon, because she was afraid that I might get her to become a vegetarian. I just shrugged my shoulders, and said that I wasn't going to lecture. Midway through the meal, her curiosity got the better of her, and she started to ask me questions. Within a week, with additional help from my copy of* Diet for a New America, *she was a vegetarian.*

Our role is not to insist, "You should become a vegetarian." There is a part within them that desires to live a healthier, more environmentally responsible, more humane life. It is already giving them that message. That is why they are conflicted! Our goal is to connect to the part of them that desires change, not the part that blocks change.

If, through their actions, people reveal they are conflicted, you cannot help their process by stuffing more information inside of them. They need to reflect on their awareness. Moreover, when you argue, or even when you are merely offering a statistic to a nonvegetarian, that statistic is associated with a voice, and that voice has a face. Our face. When they encounter a statistic on their own, the voice in their ear is their own. Awareness happens then because they aren't also trying to figure out their relationship to us *and* to the statistics.

Are you judging, angry, bitter? No matter how legitimate you believe these feelings to be, no one wants to be the recipient of someone else's unprocessed feelings. With judgment, bitterness, and inflexibility, we take on another's process. They are freed, and we become more inflexible. We often think the way to meet the intensity of someone else's emotions is with an equal intensity of emotions, fighting back, arguing. We are saying, "What about me?" "You are responsible for my feelings!"

There is an alternative. This is their issue, not ours. One cannot carry the burden of others' consciousness for them. We are trying to create the space for them to fall through their own rabbit hole into consciousness for themselves.

We need to remove ourselves. Don't step into the line of fire. Let the energy implode within the meat eater, rather than be an external agent of explosion. This explains Adams's maxim: "*Do not assume the role of superego; step out of the way if it is being projected upon you.*"

This means: Do not cause or contribute to people's anxieties about what they are eating while they are eating. Avoid statements such as: "Don't you *even* care about your health/the animals/the environment?" With such a statement, you tell them that you have the right to define exactly what caring involves. And, according to you, caring means doing what *you* are doing, not what they are doing. No one wants to hear these words, even if you are 100 percent correct. You have stated the unforgivable, causing a further separation between the two of you. You are making someone feel guilty.

Avoid, too, "*Even* a meat eater like you should know . . ." This sounds condescending, paternalistic, insulting. First, you are calling them ignorant. You are saying, in essence, "These facts are so well known, if you don't know them, you must really be ignorant. Either a) you know these facts and you are guilty of acting despite this knowledge or b) you don't know these facts and you are guilty of being ignorant."

And don't tell them that their guilt or anger is the symptom of being blocked: that will confirm that you are acting as a superego. Instead, you can say, "What matters to you is your choices, not mine. What choices are you going to make?" This reminds them that they are making choices.

People have to feel they can experiment and make mistakes without being shamed. They need a welcoming environment, not a constricted, combative one. Meat eaters do not trust vegetarians to create that space for them. In addition, meat eaters see in us a representation of what seems impossible for them: "I can't do that." "I could never do that." That makes them feel different from us. We must see in them a representation of our commonalities and do that by determining, "What in them can we connect to?"

The values that undergird our vegetarianism—values concerning health of the body and of the planet, a desire for a peaceful diet, and compassion for others—are not unique to vegetarianism. These values may be expressed by our friends in other areas of their lives where they are unblocked.

People want to be validated. Engage people with a subject you can agree on. You may agree that neglected or injured dogs should be taken care of or that heart disease or cancer is a serious concern in their lives. Much to their own surprise, they find themselves agreeing with you.

It is up to us to help nonvegetarians recognize our commonalities, not our differences. If they feel hostile or defensive, they are not going to see you as an ally, a friend. They are not going to feel that they want to become like you in their food choices.

What we can do is help them see that the process of addressing what is blocking them is a process of release from guilt, anger, and judgment. How do we do this?

We do this simply by living our vegetarian lives with ease and grace.

When we are at ease, what people sense is the absence of judgment. As a result, they are enabled to reflect for themselves, because they don't have to defend themselves from your accusations or their fears that you will accuse them. They may experience that you are at peace with yourself, and desire it for themselves. They realize that not following energy creates a lot more unhappiness and frustration than following energy: shoulda, coulda . . . *did*.

5

Sabotage and Other Meat-Eating Defenses

Meat eaters may feel miserable, but they are fairly confident that you are *more* miserable. They often try to sabotage your vegetarianism to confirm this. They successfully deflect their misery unto you. Conveniently, too, they are able to confirm for themselves that you *are* miserable. They've made you so!

"Frequently it seems as though meat eaters I know regard my choices as silly or unimportant. They seem to have this idea that I'll eat meat if it's presented in the right way, such as inviting me to dinner and providing nothing else."

"I don't like the 'joke' some meat eaters make of shoving bits of steak in my face when eating out, exclaiming, 'You really don't *want any of this?' and then laughing at my obvious disgust."*

"One of the most disturbing interactions I've had with a meat eater was in a college classroom. As the room got warmer I took off my sweatshirt to reveal an animal rights T-shirt underneath. A male student behind me nastily and loudly snapped, 'Hey, you aren't one of those vegetarian animal rights nut, are you?' When I replied that I was a vegetarian *and that I was pro-animal but not a so-called 'nut,'*

he responded by angrily telling me that after class he was going to go and get a 'nice big bloody hamburger and eat it' just for me. A few people in the class chuckled, making me feel I was being ganged up on. . . . I was so taken aback by this unprovoked assault, which was obviously intended to publicly embarrass me, that my first instinct was to tell him to enjoy his heart attack, too. However, instead I took a deep breath and asked him calmly why it was that people like him think that animal rights activists are crazed fanatics, yet it was he who shoved his beliefs, unprovoked, down my throat. Instead of reinforcing his stereotype, I called him on his own. Suddenly, he got a lot quieter and mumbled something under his breath about his not thinking animal testing for cosmetics was ethical and that he 'didn't agree' with killing animals for fur coats. . . . The 'conversation' had certainly taken an interesting turn! Since then, I've tried to keep that episode in mind when my first instinct is to return the hostility of a meat eater in kind. As an aside, ever since that incident that man would say hello every time he saw me, and even asked me out for a drink!"

When vegetarians experience sabotage, they feel hurt, confused, upset, betrayed. This chapter explores the dynamics of sabotage, what it reveals about the meat eater who engages in it, and how to protect against it. It takes the mystery out of meat eaters' actions that are hostile, hurtful, and confusing.

Saboteurs may organize their world in a very simple manner: "Well, that person is a vegetarian, they don't share my beliefs, they're bad." They also believe "if you're not for me you're against me." Such people may react strongly to you because you represent what they have failed at. They know or sense they should change, and yet they haven't. You are their negation. Your action exposes their inaction. They are watching you, hoping that you fail. Your failure is their justification. What remains for them is to create problems for you to affirm their lack of action.

Saboteurs need to believe it is too difficult to live without meat. And they help to ensure that their belief is true. They are putting a lot of energy into your vegetarianism. It is negative energy, but the very fact that they wish or are willing to put out so much energy says something. They have connected with you. Our challenge is to transform the negative into the positive.

WHAT IS SABOTAGE?

In sabotage, you experience yourself as the target of the meat eater's negative energy.

Sabotage is often the action of people who have awareness at some level that they are blocked vegetarians. They sense they "should" be vegetarian but they are not. In interacting with us, their bondage to a meat-eating culture becomes apparent. We are triggering it, but what is there—the psychological material that must be worked with—is within them. Our vegetarianism brings their bondage to their attention. The process of bringing bondage to consciousness can be very painful.

Why resort to sabotage? To block the painful process of bringing their bondage to consciousness. Acts of sabotage are the outward sign of an interior battle. Once again an interaction turns toward *us* to keep it from being about *them*. Saboteurs spend an enormous amount of energy trying to deny the integrity, legitimacy, or convenience of your choice. This is because saboteurs sense that you are right and they are wrong.

A saboteur is a boundary maintainer. Not only does the saboteur feel that with your vegetarianism the boundary is crumbling, but it is his or her efforts alone that will maintain the boundary, and you must be punished for causing its collapse. They need to believe that you cannot successfully be a vegetarian. They present obstacles to help them be convinced of this.

THE CLASSIFICATION OF SABOTEURS

The sabotage dynamic arises from a drive for power and a need to eliminate/vanquish that which threatens. Saboteurs may be the group most truly threatened by your vegetarianism. That's the last thing they can admit to themselves or to you. Saboteurs may also get secret and not-so-secret pleasure from causing difficulty. By erecting barriers to your vegetarianism, they forcefully prove to themselves that vegetarianism is just too hard to accomplish.

Saboteurs lead with their insecurity about themselves and their diet. Whenever people lead with their insecurity, we should recognize that they are feeling threatened. They put it explicitly out on the table for us to examine. How helpful of them, really!

The "Caring" Saboteur

Caring saboteurs hide their actions. Outwardly they are charismatic, charming, attentive, caring . . . to a degree. Caring saboteurs would never see themselves as saboteurs. They care about you; they wouldn't deliberately hurt you or frustrate you!

Caring saboteurs promise to give you food that you can eat. But they don't deliver. You get chicken broth in the soup or egg in the dessert, and their pronouncement that something is vegetarian or vegan when it isn't. A caring saboteur knows precisely what you do and don't eat; this is not the casual host who is unaware. They deliberately deviate from what you can eat. They rationalize it one way or another. They can't change, but they don't want to admit it. At least not in advance. They want to wait until the etiquette required of you as a guest at dinner prevents too much prying into their motivations. So they don't tell the vegetarian in advance that they didn't vary their cooking methods, though they had offered to prepare food the vegetarian could eat. They act as though they understand and will respect your food boundaries, but in fact they don't because they can't. Their excuse might be: *I know you said that you don't eat eggs, but really it's the only way this dessert could be made and I figured you wouldn't mind this once.* (They rarely have to articulate their excuse, however, because we are constrained by politeness not to criticize them.) What they are really saying is, "I can't let your decision matter. I have to punish you for your decision. I don't care enough about you to meet you here. But I don't want to know I am really this uncaring." Or, more aggressively, but still not explicitly: "I'll show you the only way I can. You think you are going to get me to think about your dietary needs in advance? Well, I simply refuse to. If I think about your dietary needs in advance, that would mean I could think about mine in advance." But, of course, they *are* thinking about it in advance, thinking about how to indicate that they are *not* thinking about it. They must block awareness—yours, by thwarting your vegetarianism, and their own, by manifesting their refusal to engage with the issue.

I am not talking here about superficial acquaintances or dinner parties where you don't know the host, all those interactions that bring us into the sphere of people we don't know well. I am talking about friends, good friends, people we enjoy being with, people who we think care about us. This is the crunch. In practically every other way that they interact with us, they *are* caring. We feel embraced by them. Yet when it comes to our food differences, we experience something else entirely. We are invited to brunch and the margarine we left at their house so that we could have something on our bagels has disappeared. We are invited to dinner and they confess, "Well, I did put some chicken broth in the ratatouille."

What are we to do? The caring saboteur requires some special attention that other kinds of saboteurs might not. We are connected to the caring saboteur in ways that complicate our responses. Yet, really, all that is required of you is to make explicit what is being promised. That way you have a foundation for judging whatever happens next. For instance, the caring saboteur offers to make something. Say it is the dessert for the yearly holiday celebration that you share with them. Maybe it is a vegan cake. To confirm precisely what the cake will contain, you could pursue the issue in this gentle way:

> You: "I'm looking forward to our yearly dinner. It will be very nice."
> Host: "Yes, I am, too."
> You: "What kind of cake are you making?"

> *Host: "A Meyer lemon cake."*
> *You: "That sounds great!"*

Then, you follow that up immediately with a question such as "Where did you find a Meyer lemon cake recipe that doesn't use eggs?" or "What egg substitute do you like best?" Or, even more explicitly, if they understand what the word *vegan* entails: "Where did you find a vegan lemon cake recipe?"

Through this conversation, you make explicit that the person is promising an eggless cake. Of course, the dish in question might be a meatless moussaka or a tofu quiche. It does not matter what is being offered; what matters is to *clarify* that they are offering to prepare something that respects your dietary commitments. This assures you of their awareness of what they are promising and gives them an out if this is not what they are really promising.

If, after clarifying what has been promised, you are still presented with a cake with eggs in it, a moussaka with meat in it, or a traditional quiche, you know that the failure was deliberate and not an oversight. This is information you need to know. It will probably prompt a reevaluation of the relationship. Because what they are saying to you is: "You are not as important to me as you thought." Why is that? What is never acknowledged, but may be underlying the sabotage, is: "I cannot allow myself to care about your diet. There is something painful for me if I connect to your veganism without being a vegan. I can't admit this to myself, much less to you." But, as a result, they are also telling you that you need to say to yourself: "Here is someone I can't trust. This person is not able to respect something central to my life. In the future, I need to be alert to this." After that, no matter what they promise, do not expect that they are really able to feed you, no matter how much they may think they want to. Eat before you go or bring a second dessert just for the fun of it.

The *parental* caring saboteur is concerned that one cannot actually survive without meat, so she or he puts meat or dairy in your food but doesn't tell you. The mother of one young woman fed her eggs cooked in bacon. Only when the daughter got ill did the mother stop doing this. One father stuffs meat into his daughter's food when she goes to the bathroom or is away from the table. If you are in this situation, make sure your parents have an opportunity to read Appendix B, "Letter to Parents of Vegetarians."

A final subset of the caring saboteur are "false allies." They exhibit some enthusiasm, but it's fake, only to get you softened up for the insult that is coming. They have to first empower themselves by getting themselves trusted, only to hurt you the more. Not much can be done in defense of these saboteurs, because by the time you realize what has happened, it is too late: you let your guard down and they have used your trust to hurt you. They are not only blocked vegetarians but untrustworthy ones at that.

The Dominance and Control Saboteur

Upon learning that you are vegetarian, people may change their own eating habits, but not necessarily in a positive direction. They may feel challenged to express their meat eating. Where they used to eat meat without much consciousness, they must now proclaim themselves eager and happy meat eaters. Sometimes they take on an air of belligerence, pronouncedly eating meat in front of you as an attempt to disgust or upset you. It is actually an attempt to establish control over the situation.

A friend may announce, "I want the cow brought right here, so I can butcher it myself!" or "We want the juicy flesh burgers!" Meat is the vehicle for them to reestablish some control over the situation, a situation in which they are profoundly defensive.

This saboteur often assumes that he or she is interacting with a "Bambi vegetarian." He or she declares in words and actions, "I know I am eating animals. I am proud of it! I'm strong enough to eat this once-living animal with no effect on my conscience!" This saboteur has a problem with feelings. "Bambi vegetarians" are seen as people who lead with their emotions. Of course, the motivations around responding to animal suffering are much more complex than this simplistic formula. But an individual who treats feelings with ridicule and irony will treat those people who represent feelings—vegetarians—with ridicule and irony. They declare to all and sundry: "This shows how much in control of myself I am, that I knowingly eat a dead animal." They provide reassurance that they and their culture have chosen the right way.

What is underneath the bluff, the bravado? People who are afraid to care, people who are afraid to change. Which means they have the potential to care and the potential to change. Their reactions announce that they are blocking their energy. There is a part of them that wishes to change. You remind them of that part.

They simply need reassurance that feelings don't destroy one, that feelings can be integrated within a healthy, functioning adult. Of course, you may not be what meat eaters reductively call a "Bambi vegetarian." You may have become a vegetarian for another reason entirely. It does not matter to these saboteurs what your motivations are; what matters is what is unresolved within them.

Often a dominance and control saboteur requires an audience to ennoble his or her comments. Many of my correspondents reported that attacks were conducted among groups. Acting out with others present emboldens these saboteurs. They don't have to argue about facts or issues; they can simply intimidate or ridicule and hope that others go along or don't call them on it.

What should you do in the face of the dominance and control saboteur? The opposite of being annoyed is to *ignore*. Ignore their negative energy. Ignoring is an active process of responding to conflicting emotions and not letting them overwhelm you. Don't get worked up. You can turn to them and say simply, "That was unkind." You aren't being defensive or argumentative, and by noting their behavior you give a reason for ignoring them. Or you can say, "That wasn't a very nice thing to do." Then, make a *third*-person observation that is not directly threatening to the audience: "Many people find vegetarians threatening because there is a part of them that wants to avoid animal flesh for a lot of good reasons, but another part doesn't want to stop eating meat."

You can demonstrate concern and caring, while refusing to accept the saboteur's agenda, with an "I wonder" response. For example: "I wonder what animals in slaughterhouses feel like. They certainly seem terrified." Or, "I wonder what would happen if people consumed less meat. I wonder if it would free up grains to feed malnourished people."

In this, you reveal that feelings do not destroy. You demonstrate a form of emotional strength, not through control but through awareness.

The Hostile Saboteur

These constitute a very nervous subset of the dominance and control saboteur. But they fill up the vegetarian's eating space so frequently and obnoxiously that we need to consider them as a separate species of meat eaters. Through several predictable tactics, hostile saboteurs hyperinflate meat's importance at a meal.

The first tactic is to provide a narration of their meal. I call this "eating out loud." The hostile saboteur acts out his fears of giving up meat by calling attention to meat eating. "Hmmmmm, I love meat *so* much! Watch as I bite into this burger and blood drips down the side of my mouth."

One vegetarian described a meal with someone who was eating out loud:

> At my company's last Christmas luncheon, one meat eater in partic-
> ular chose to tell the table about every piece of seafood from the gumbo
> that he was eating—first, I told him that I didn't want a play-by-
> play of his meal, and then as he continued I chimed in and did a play-
> by-play of my veggie stir-fry—look at this broccoli, wow, what a
> mushroom, etc. The table got a laugh and he finally shut up, so it
> worked out well.

Her co-worker is exhibiting fear. He is latching on to every bite he thinks she will take away from him, and taunting her with his intensified attachment. But what is he really saying? "You, sitting there eating your veggie stir-fry, make me so uneasy about meat eating that I must protect it, and accompany my actions with words." Eating out loud happens because someone feels his attachment is being threatened. He is trying to provide security for himself by providing a bite-by-bite narrative. How secure, actually, is his meat eating if one lone vegetarian eating her veggie stir-fry can evoke such defensive behavior?

Another tactic is to bring meat into your personal space. I call these saboteurs "meat thrusters." Waving, say, a pepperoni pizza or a hamburger in front of you—or whatever they are eating—they say, "Come on. You know you get the urge to have some meat. You know you want some of this." Thrusters take a taunting approach, trying to "break you" of your vegetarianism while also trying to have their meal validated by you.

I used to work with a guy who would always tease me with his meat sandwich. He would stick it in my face and say, "Come on, you know you want it. Dead flesh is so good, mmmm!" I never argued with him about it and usually I would just smile and continue to eat my lunch. Then one day he wanted to try something I had brought for lunch, and he liked it. From that day on he was always curious to know what I was eating, and I intentionally started bringing more food because I knew he would want some. After exciting his taste buds for several weeks, he confessed that he had cut back on eating meat, and he wondered if I had any info on vegetarianism that I could share with him. A well-armed vegetarian always has an arsenal of information at all times. I gave him Dr. Michael Klaper's video A Diet for All Reasons. *He came back to me the next day and said, "That's it, I'm never eating meat again." I was pretty shocked because he was a big meat eater. Today this friend is one of the most committed vegetarians I know.*

This vegetarian understood the necessity of ignoring a meat thruster. By ignoring that energy, the space was provided for the meat eater to begin to change. How do you cultivate the ability to ignore?

Simply follow the rules of etiquette: Don't respond to their offensive behavior and instead repeat the mantra of "No thanks. No thank you. . . . No thank you."

The final subset of the dominance and control saboteur is the *diluter*. The diluter wants to dilute, minimize, and reduce consciousness about animals by applying the vegetarian's concern to everything under the sun. The diluter will pick up a flower, or take a branch, and say, "Aren't you worried about the little plant?" or "Oh, I hear those vegetables crying." Bugs will suddenly become objects of concern. The attempt is to restrict through dilution the power of the vegetarian's implicit message. Of course, many vegetarians are concerned about plants and bugs, but this is probably not the time to discuss a nonviolent eating ethic. One teenager described this form of joking that greeted her vegetarianism. At some point, she realized, these people were making fun of her to make themselves look better. Again the rules of etiquette apply here: Always be respectful. Your critic is a conflicted, suffering, blocked vegetarian.

Now the question might arise: When a saboteur makes you feel uncomfortable, awkward, or humiliated, why can't you simply respond by telling them off or arguing with them? Because this feeds them. This is what they want. This allows them to become self-righteous, and that is their coping mechanism against their own fragmented consciousness.

A certain moral superiority is derived from lampooning, gossiping about, or criticizing someone who is doing something that makes you inwardly uneasy. For the dominance and control saboteur your choice has to be made unworthy, negative; it has to lose any of its attraction. They will exploit whatever they can—your uptightness, your tofu, your lack of a sense of humor—to maintain control. All of this criticism and cruelty show that some people are working mighty hard to maintain their sense of the acceptability of meat eating. This is actually a good sign! The greater their disturbance, the harder it is for them to reclaim that acceptability.

The Boundary-Keeping Saboteur

Boundary-keeping saboteurs use accusations to make you insecure, hoping that feelings of insecurity and peer pressure will bring you into line. They are enforcers of the status quo. Conformity is the issue.

Many of the teenagers I talked with felt that other teenagers were less tolerant than adults were of their vegetarianism. They felt that teenagers were less flexible in accepting differences.

Often boundary-keeping saboteurs try to enforce conformity by using the gender issues of the culture. They will accuse males who are vegetarian of being gay. They accept the idea that men need meat, and so when a man doesn't eat meat it means that he is not comfortable being "male," according to their conventional definition. Combine that with a lack of sophistication about sexuality, and the conclusion is that the male in question is gay. "You're a pansy [fruit, fairy], you don't eat meat."

Boundary keepers will similarly accuse females who are vegetarian of being lesbians. "I was in high school and the boys found out I was a vegetarian. They responded by calling me a lesbian." Boundary-keeping saboteurs use questions of sexuality that are acutely alive at this time in their lives to bring other forms of perceived deviance into line. Boundary keepers are defensive about your vegetarianism. In their actions, they are betting that you are defensive about your sexual identity. Again, the way to respond is simply to ignore them or smile at them.

The "Vegetarian" Saboteur

Many vegetarians have had the experience of discovering that some omnivores who do not eat four-legged animals have preceded them to a restaurant and, calling themselves "vegetarian," ordered chicken or fish. Thus they teach everyone they interact with that a vegetarian eats dead animals. When an actual vegetarian enters that same restaurant, or eats with the same friends who have been exposed to the faux vegetarian, you are the one who will suffer. These faux "vegetarians" are ruining our ability to assume anything about anyone when the issue is vegetarianism. So, first, don't assume, ever, that anyone understands what you mean when you say that you are a vegetarian. Be explicit. "I am a vegetarian. I don't eat anything with a face" (or, "anything with eyes except potatoes" or, "anything that had a mother"). Second, contain the faux vegetarian's damage, in this way—enclose "vegetarian" in quotation marks. By doing so you problematize their definition without getting all worked up: "Oh, you must have entertained one of those quote unquote vegetarians who think chicken and fish grow on trees." And if you meet anyone who calls herself vegetarian even though she fails to adhere to a vegetarian diet, don't get into an argument, just assume she is misinformed. Offer to send her some information about vegetarianism. Vegan Outreach publishes two helpful pamphlets, *Why Vegan?* and *Vegetarian Living*. It will be clear from these writings why chickens and fish are not part of a vegetarian diet. Let them encounter the fact for themselves and, in doing so, derive the benefits of self-reflection. These actions are ways of restoring the appropriate definition and of restoring our equilibrium at the same time. In the meantime, don't assume that calling yourself a vegetarian will convey anything accurate to others about what you do or don't eat.

WHY DO MEAT EATERS SABOTAGE VEGETARIANS?

Because meat eaters live among meat eaters and have their world reflected back to them, their understanding of a vegetarian life is impoverished. They relate to you from that impoverishment. The result is that they cause vegetarians to feel momentarily impoverished—by not preparing food that we could eat when they promised they would or creating a most unwelcome environment for our meals.

When a vegetarian sits down to eat with another person, that person's choice of food may become obvious. In our presence, they recognize that they are meat eaters. What are they going to do with that recognition? Saboteurs take the defensiveness they feel about this fact and magnify it, manifest it, act it out against us. They have a lot of dynamic life energy. They have not learned how to channel it positively.

87

Saboteurs discount your reality and violate your needs. Something fairly urgent must be at work in them for them to act in such duplicitous, unkind, often cruel, or obnoxious ways. These people fear becoming vegetarians themselves. Sharon Salzberg observes, "Fear can often give rise to an intensified attachment, because if we fear that something might be taken away, we will crave for a means to secure it."

The saboteur may also feel insecurity: "I'm being judged and found inadequate. Well, I'll show them." They want you to take on their unwanted feelings so they transfer their discomfort to you. Through sabotage their outer actions mirror their interior crisis—they are sabotaging their own best desires, for lack of something: lack of courage to change, lack of sense of safety to change. We may not be privy to the specifics, but we experience the behavior.

So much of a barrier, so much resistance, announce that something is there. This means they have the potential to change. Not only that: you are triggering something inside them because of that potential, which they must actively quiet by turning their inner torment on you.

The saboteur is internally conflicted. Through sabotage, they bring this conflict outward and let you carry it for them.

THE RESULTS OF RESPONDING WITH ABUNDANCE

In Chapter 2, "Are You at Peace?" I suggested that meat eaters view vegetarians as choosing scarcity in the face of a meat-eating world's abundance. Sabotage at one level is an attempt by a meat eater to inflict this distorted scarcity model upon you. They confirm their fears that living without meat is living without food choices by acting them out *against* you.

When you are unperturbed by sabotage, when you continue to enjoy your meal and refuse to engage with the saboteur's negative energy, you demonstrate a sense of abundance in relationship to your own meal. By ignoring their rude and cruel behavior, you show that vegetarianism is so positive that it neutralizes their negative energy. By continuing to respond positively, you demonstrate a sense of abundance.

They need to believe that living without meat can't happily be done, even though they are the cause of the unhappiness. Of course it is irrational, but that doesn't keep them from trying to sabotage you. Because this need to inflict the distorted scarcity model they have for vegetarianism upon you is irrational, you can't simply reassure them by saying, "It's okay. Being a vegetarian is fine!" Rather than telling them anything, you have to let your actions speak on your behalf. They need to experience something that words cannot impart—that your vegetarianism is so transformative, they and their negative energy can't disrupt it, destroy it, diminish it. They need to see before them someone who is not disturbed by their actions. Then they *see* from your behavior that being a vegetarian is fine. You convey this in these often toughest of interactions simply by continuing to enjoy your choice of foods, no matter how restricted those choices are at that moment.

Saboteurs are making the best choices available in their model of the world. Their model says, "Meat and dairy are necessary [for me to feel happy/full/healthy]!" So they choose accordingly. The thing is not to challenge the choices they make but to change the model. When you continue to express your sense of abundance, despite their actions, you undermine their fears of scarcity. "It is nothing," you say. "No big deal." You are happy with your choices.

We challenge this notion of vegetarianism as impoverishment by living a life that expresses a sense of abundance. "Oh, you put eggs in that cake? I guess I'll wait for dessert later." No big deal. This sense of abundance is contagious.

The most obnoxious nonvegetarians spend so much time trying to thwart you that they end up studying you. Some of the grossest violators of manners, meat thrusters, often become the ones touched by the vegetarian's unperturbed responses and enjoyment of their food. They discover, "While I am miserable, vegetarians, contrary to my thoughts, are not more miserable. They are considerably *less* miserable."

Sometimes those who badger or antagonize are actually the most interested in your diet; their defensive behavior is an attempt to protect them from their own leanings. Those who may be the biggest offenders—the ones who shove meat in your face and those who eat out loud—might be defending themselves the most strongly from what they have themselves come to sense about meat eating: it isn't necessary. The greater the doubt and the greater the criticism, the greater the attraction and the greater the possibility.

How ironic! Saboteurs may be the most likely vegetarian converts, and sabotage is their final barricade against change! How can we tell? The clue is the intensity of energy with which they respond to your vegetarianism.

The saboteur is the most likely to change because, at some level, the saboteur perceives the fluidity of change: that one can leave meat eating and become a vegetarian. The saboteur recoils from such a fate. She or he does not want change, even fluid, natural, evolving change, to work its magic on him or her. Sabotage is the Berlin Wall of psychic defensiveness: it keeps the saboteur seemingly safe from change.

But Berlin Walls fall, and as the saboteur continues to hang around, what do you know . . . they become vegetarians! I've heard that story over and over again from vegetarians.

How did you become a vegetarian?

The ex-saboteur's answer: I watched a vegetarian live her life.

6

Talking with Meat Eaters

Two kinds of people exist in the world: those who want answers to their questions and those who don't. More important than knowing the answers to questions is having the skill to tell the difference between these people.

Conversations may be one way that meat eaters learn about vegetarianism; but they are also the most stubborn way that meat eaters hold on to their lifestyle. Indeed, conversations themselves are functioning differently for meat eaters than for vegetarians. Frequently, meat eaters are trying to find ways to dull the impact of our words, while we are constantly finding ways to sharpen those words.

Numerous vegetarian organizations, books, and Web sites provide definitive answers to every possible question a meat eater might throw at a vegetarian. "Be prepared," these answers suggest. They imply, "If you are prepared, your conversations will be easier, less stressful." The intentions of these answers to frequently asked questions are admirable, but they misunderstand a basic dynamic: *You cannot argue with a people's mythology.*

Meat eating is one of our culture's mythologies. Atlas will fling the world off his shoulders before we dislodge this mythology through argument alone. Moreover, the questions meat eaters *ask* may not be the questions meat eaters *need answered*. Often, the content of the conversation itself is the least important aspect of a conversation. You need to learn how to identify the question behind the question.

You should assume that for the meat eater, conversations with you function to distort and block your perspective as much as they function to convey information. This perspective accounts for my basic rules for talking with meat eaters.

Basic Rules for Talking with Meat Eaters

1. Don't discuss vegetarianism while people are eating meat and dairy. At a nonverbal level, contents of the meal disempower the vegetarian while making meat eaters more defensive. One can simply state, "I'm glad to talk about vegetarianism, because it's very important to me. But I find that it can spoil my appetite to talk about eating meat over meals. Let's discuss this later."

2. Less is more. Or, "Here I am, come to me." Rather than feeling that we have to show, to demonstrate, to vindicate ourselves or vegetarianism, see all interactions as a process of coming to consciousness.

3. Don't feel that you need to answer any or every question. Instead, order multiple copies of *Why Vegan?* and *Vegetarian Living* and hand them out. (Each is sixteen pages long and available from Vegan Outreach, 211 Indian Drive, Pittsburgh, PA 15328; 412-968-0268; Info@vegliving.org or www.vegliving.org.) A lengthier, more eclectic, but equally compelling pamphlet is *101 Reasons Why I'm a Vegetarian* by Pamela Rice (available from VivaVeggie Society, P.O. Box 294, Prince Street Station, New York, NY 10012). Choose a pamphlet that best represents your viewpoint or is the most appropriate one for your interlocutor.

4. Speak to meat eaters the way you would speak to a wild animal: softly and without any sudden movements.

5. If you are going to have a conversation with a person, the first statement you make should indicate some sort of agreement with the person: "Yes, that's an interesting point." Then you might say, "Many people don't know that . . ." This allows you to provide information in

a way that is not confrontational or condescending. For example: "Many people don't know that animals on farms suffer greatly from crowded, stressful conditions and manipulations. I choose not to contribute to that. I wonder what else people can do, short of becoming vegetarian."

6. In a social context, it is wise never to try to encourage someone to change diets.

7. If you ignore rule no. 1, or are repeatedly pulled into a mealtime exchange, continually take the pulse of the conversation (see pages 120–121) so that you can end it if you need to.

What accounts for these rules and my pessimistic view of the function of conversations? My understanding of the vegetarian–meat eater conversational divide.

THE VEGETARIAN–MEAT EATER CONVERSATIONAL DIVIDE

Say you have just been asked, in mixed company, "So, tell me: Why are you a vegetarian?"

You say, "I'd rather not talk about it while you are eating."

"No, really, why did you become a vegetarian?"

After several attempts to postpone an answer, you give in. "The ribs I stared at on my plate looked just like the cadaver I faced the week before as a medical school student."

Or, you might talk about how you realized the relationship between meat and dairy consumption and heart attacks. You are being honest. But you are also being literal. You are talking about animals' bodies.

Speaking Literally

Vegetarians have a tendency to speak literally; our culture avoids the literal. We vegetarians say meat is *muscle* from a *corpse* or eggs are reproductive secretions. While literal thinking is important in understanding the world, literal thinking can also trip us up, especially when the issue is animal exploitation. As I point out in *The Sexual Politics of Meat,* part of the battle of being heard as a vegetarian is being heard about literal matters in a society that favors euphemistic expressions.

You are asked, "Why are you a vegetarian?" And you say, "I just don't want to eat dead animals." Or, "I think of meat as an animal's corpse."

Suddenly the nonvegetarians—thinking that they were engaging in nothing more than a pleasant "get to know you" question—find that the conversation has changed in intensity. By answering honestly about what you have learned about meat eating and dairy production/consumption—factual information—you are prompting a connection in the nonvegetarian with something they have usually blocked out of their consciousness. Suddenly, somewhere in themselves, a part of them says, "Whoa! What's happening here? I don't want to hear this information! This makes me feel uncomfortable. Who is that person to make me feel uncomfortable? Oh, those emotional vegetarians."

Literal speech is experienced emotionally.

You stated a literal truth or fact. It is experienced as an emotional statement because its content prompts feelings within the nonvegetarian, feelings the nonvegetarian does not want to be aware of. You will very shortly thereafter be accused of being emotional.

Translating a Foreign Language

We know a lot more about meat eating than most meat eaters. This is probably one of the reasons we became vegetarians. We don't have to resist this information. We aren't blocked. The problem is that *the person with the least amount of information sets the level of the conversation.* If the person with the least amount of information sets the level of the conversation, control is automatically vested with the meat eater.

Here's an example: when Ronald Reagan was president, he had to meet with François Mitterrand, then president of France. Reagan spoke

English; Mitterrand, French and English. Which language did they speak? English, of course.

Meat eaters speak one language. Vegetarians speak two. Among ourselves, we might exchange tofu and tempeh recipes, discuss how to veganize a recipe, make plans to go to a vegetarian restaurant, or attend a protest against factory farms. We are speaking "French." Among meat eaters—"English speakers"—we have to translate constantly from French into English. Ask any translator—this is hard work! This is not how we relax. What is inherent in our experience, what is integrated, has to be pried apart to explain to someone else.

You do not have to teach them the language. Instead, get their e-mail address, fax number, or snail mail address. Send them your favorite fact sheet (such as *Why Vegan?*, *Vegetarian Living*, or *101 Reasons Why I'm a Vegetarian* [see page 92]) and a few of your favorite recipes.

Just the Facts?

Remember, if you reel off statistics, the voice in their mind will be yours. If for no other reason, you should resist reciting facts, although it may be your first instinct. Vegetarians look as if they are trying to be experts when they use statistics. Many people distrust anyone who throws facts at them. It's not conversational. They may feel lectured at. Most meat eaters don't want vegetarians to be experts. Moreover, people distrust facts. They are suspicious. How have we manipulated the facts? Who compiled them? How do we know they are true? You are seen as someone with a point to get across, you are not seen as unbiased and fair.

Another problem with facts is that the numbers we might cite about the implications of meat eating are simply too big to be comprehended. Innumeracy—mathematical illiteracy—works in favor of meat eating. The Greek mathematician Archimedes pointed out that a bunch of small numbers when added together will exceed any large number, no matter how great it is. Of course he said it more elegantly than this.

This "additivity" of small numbers explains how 200 pounds of meat per person per year translates to over 9 billion land animals. If one doesn't grasp the additivity of small numbers, he or she won't see how his or her individual role as a meat eater contributes to global warming, deforestation, and the deaths of so many animals.

Remember that dispersing facts may also play into the meat eater's need to keep this controlled and rational, because they are trying to keep themselves controlled and rational.

The Right Brain–Left Brain Divide

Questions from meat eaters may arise as a way to avoid their own feelings. Regardless of the content, talking becomes a defensive mechanism in and of itself. They are working so hard to keep the left brain in control. They have to prevent any sort of associations that might pull their right brain in. So they keep things linear and controlled. How? By following the basic format of question-and-answer. Many meat eaters are already thinking of their next argument while you answer the one they have just given you. It is not really a conversation; it is a stalling technique. And the questions will be ones that overintellectualize, such as, "What if you were stranded on a desert island and all you had to eat was a snake?" They want to know how you have anticipated every contingency. Are you going to make exceptions or not? What vegetarian doesn't hate these questions? One response is to say, "I'll decide about that then, but it's not relevant to my situation here, today." Of course, honoring the question keeps the focus on you and postpones any self-examination for them. You might not want to do this.

Here is another overintellectualized question: "What is the vegetarian vision for twenty years from now?" Should we answer that question? Most of us probably could, by rattling off ideas about reduction or elimination of meat eating, less heart attacks, environmental health, etc. This is not the point. The meat eater, on two separate levels, is keeping distance from the issue. First, by thinking he needs to have everything mapped out, as though it is *this* vision that will make him more open to vegetarianism. It is a way of postponing dealing with his own role in meat eating. You can say, "Who knows? But I haven't eaten meat in [X] years and I'm not going to eat any today." Recognize, however, that the question itself announces that the status quo is at work. Why do vegetarians have to have a plan, but meat eaters don't?

How could you answer this question in such a way that the meat eater isn't allowed to keep postponing? By asking a question back:

What is the meat eater's plan for twenty years from now?
Why, given the issues today, is that important to you?
What interests you about vegetarianism today?

Drastic questions such as "If everyone became a vegetarian overnight, what would happen to all the animals?" tell us that people feel that vegetarianism is drastic for them personally. They externalize this feeling in their questions. If they only thought about it for a minute, they would realize they are asking about an impossibility.

Watch out for a conversation in which a meat eater announces, "My vegetarian friends don't have an answer for this" before asking the question. Of course, he is creating a greater burden on the vegetarian—and tempting you, too. We might presume, "Oh, if I can answer *this* question, I will convince him." When I hear this I know:

1. He has argued and pursued issues with other vegetarians. I am not the first; I won't be the last.
2. He was happy they couldn't answer the question. As long as there is no answer to the question, he doesn't have to deal with vegetarianism. He is putting the bar for vegetarianism at a level that would be difficult for it to meet. Meanwhile, he is protected from thinking about meat eating.
3. He is avoiding emotional work. He wants to control the questions and his own consciousness. The right brain–left brain problem is his.

If you want to continue a discussion with someone who is this resistant, you might do it in this manner:

"It seems to me that most opponents of vegetarianism seem threatened by this diet. Do you find it threatening?" The likely response is "No." Then, "Why don't you become a vegetarian?" "Because I like meat." Pause, with pensive look, and say, "So . . . it sounds like you are worried that you will miss the taste of meat." This is rather nonjudgmental—just an observation. Yet it identifies the problem as being with them, not with you.

STRATEGIES FOR CONVERSATIONS

Etiquette Rules!

Be aware of the basic rules for etiquette and follow them. "Why are you a vegetarian?" is a personal question and you have the right not to answer it. When someone is treating you rudely, you have the right not to answer them. You can say simply, "That's personal. I'd prefer not to talk about this at the moment."

Use a Conversational Thermometer: Is Their Question Hot, Neutral, or Cold?

A hot question often reveals anger, suppressed hostility. Examples include:

"Why are you wearing leather?"
"What about plants?"
"Hitler was a vegetarian. What do you have to say about that?"

Hot questions challenge. They keep the focus on you and vegetarianism. "Hot" questions want to put you in the hot seat. They are

ostensibly neutral, or academic. But they are not. They are confronta-
tive, argumentative.

You do not need to answer a hot question. In fact, you should avoid
it. Again, get their address and tell them you will send them some information. Your motivation here is to require them to put a little more
effort into learning about vegetarianism than simply exhausting a vegetarian with their defensive questions.

You can say, "I can see you have some interest in the topic. But I
make it a practice not to discuss vegetarianism when I am [eating/work-
ing/walking/making love/first getting to know someone . . .]. Let me
send you some information." In this way, you refuse to be a victim of
a blocked vegetarian.

What is blocking them? A "cold" question or comment tells you.
It explains why they are frozen.

> It's too hard!
> I could never do that!
> Don't you miss meat?

It's okay to follow a "cold" statement. You do so by asking questions back instead of giving answers:

> Why do you think it's too hard?
> Why do you think you couldn't?
> Are you afraid you would miss meat?

If they ask you, "Don't you ever miss a cheeseburger?" you might
respond: "No. But people ask me questions like that all the time. I wonder if they are really thinking that they would miss cheeseburgers if they
chose to be vegetarians. I don't know, but I can tell you that I thought
I might miss meat, but when I found out about [X] I realized that I had
to be a vegetarian, and I haven't regretted the choice." Or you can say,
as my friend Sarah does, "Sometimes I miss pork chops and eel sushi,

but when I stop to think about what pork and eel are made of, I know that I don't want to put that in my body."

A hot question highlights the differences between the nonvegetarian and vegetarian. The gap widens. A cold question allows the vegetarian, if they wish to pursue it, to make a bridge—to help meat eaters feel less different.

Neutral questions are elusive to pinpoint. Much in a conversation is ostensibly neutral, but because of the complex psychological mechanism that keeps someone blocked, anything that begins neutrally may quickly heat up. After all, meat eaters don't even recognize that the seemingly neutral question "Why are you a vegetarian?" will quickly heat up a conversation if it is answered. What you might see as a neutral answer will be experienced as "hot" to the meat eater. It is hot because they feel judged.

"How do you get your protein?" is a neutral question.

Answering a neutral question is fine, as long as it stays neutral. Giving information in a neutral tone allows the meat eater an opportunity to hear. Here is how one person goes about it:

I explain in a very even tone my reasons for my choices: ethics, health, and the environment. I tell them that I was a voracious meat eater for twenty-four years before I was exposed to life-changing information. I also tell them that I do not judge people based on their eating habits because I myself was on the other side, and if they would like to know more I would love to give them more information.

You need to maintain the neutrality of the question in your answer and deny people the opportunity to use your behavior to start an argument.

Look to Their Bodies

Of course meat eaters are going to respond with their bodies. We eat with our bodies! We look, smell, taste. It is only common sense that the body will register reactions as well.

We have to develop the ability to listen to their bodies as well as their words. Otherwise, we may answer the wrong questions. Body language may be telling you more than verbal content.

- Do they furrow their brows, raise their eyebrows with a bemused, skeptical smile? Show distrust of your words by recoiling from you?
- Are their arms across the chest, closing the person off, protecting them from (verbal) blows?
- Are they smiling, or not?
- Are you smiling? Is it a deferential, "I'll-try-not-to-disturb-you" smile? Are you nervous, eager to please?
- Are they breathing rapidly?
- Is their chin jutted out? Or their shoulders scrunched?
- What is happening with their eyes; are they narrowed or wide open?
- Is the tempo of their speech rapid?
- Is their tone shrill?

These are defensive postures.

Are you receiving a conflicting message from a meat eater? They say, "I am interested," but their body is rigid, and they are grimacing. Or "Tell me more," they say, yet their fists are clenched and their body stiffens as they lean away from you. They are communicating to you that they are not really interested. They are actually conflicted. They cannot bring all of themselves to the interaction.

Are they listening? Are they responding? Listen to their bodies before you answer that next question of theirs.

Use a Lighthearted Tone

Be aware of your tone. You need to convey through your speaking dynamics that you are at peace. Keep calm. Don't raise your voice. Smile, listen calmly, and nod at what they have to say. Rephrase and repeat back to them what they said. This demonstrates that you have heard and understood them.

Being playful is important. Resist the temptation to preach. People want question marks, not exclamation points ("It's better for you!" "Think about the animals!"). They want to be asked, "How do you feel?", not told, "This is how you should feel!".

This is an ironic time. Nothing is to be taken too seriously. If you take something too seriously you are immediately suspect. Vegetarians are perceived as being too earnest. Your earnestness, in and of itself, may provide meat eaters with a target outside themselves upon which to focus their anger, frustration, or disappointment with themselves. You believe. You are sure. They are uncomfortable and unsure. Irony speaks to them in their discomfort. They wish to distance themselves from your earnestness, which they can experience as tediousness. You have to relate with lightheartedness, too.

You have to find ways to displace earnestness with a shrugging nonchalance. You can be ironically dismissive, as in, "I won't tell you about the relationship between meat eating and six out of the ten diseases that kill Americans." But in saying that you *won't* tell them, you *do* tell them, and this way you do it with a wink.

When a Meat Eater Is Hostile, Pick a One-Liner and Stick to It

Decide what you wish to say about being a vegetarian and simply repeat it. Refuse to answer any other question.

"Geez, it's not like I gave up chocolate or anything!"
"I want my diet to be animal free."
"I don't think animals should have to die to give me life."
"I am healthier."
"Anything that lived or breathed isn't my idea of food."
"Life is too precious to take unnecessarily."

"My vegetarianism is part of the process of being honest with
   myself."

"This is how it is with me. I am happy."

"I do what I have to to sleep at night."

"I don't eat food from an animal that had a face, a mother, or
   a bowel movement."

"Look, I am not forcing this on you, so there is no reason for
   disrespect."

"I can't think of a reason not to."

They respond, "But what about [X]?"

Ignore whatever they put forth. Stick to your one-liner. You can
say, "I have nothing more to say." And then repeat your one-liner.
Whatever the statement is, simply repeat it over and over again, being
sure not to interrupt. Don't sound haughty in repeating it, simply
make it a statement of fact. Don't put an extra stress on any of the
words. The person may think that you can't answer their arguments. It
doesn't matter. They may taunt you: "Is that all you have to say?"
Remember: They are trying to draw you into their drama with meat
eating. You don't have to say, "I don't want to explain myself." Your
answer says it. Remember, too, that you can offer to send them literature or carry it with you.

One-Liner Answers to Typical Meat-Eaters'
Questions or Defenses

Okay, now, I am not really advising that you do this frequently. You will
be seen as hostile and uncooperative, and will allow the meat eater to
control the conversation and avoid dealing with their own role in meat
eating. But everyone needs some variety, and so do we vegetarians.
Sometimes, you might feel that you need to answer some of the
defenses that are flung at you in the meat eater's desperate move to stay
blocked. Here are some one-liners to fling back:

They: "Yes, well, it's a dog-eat-dog world."
You: "No one is eating us."
Or
You: "In fact, it isn't. Only five percent of all animals are killed by other animals."

They: "This is part of our animal nature."
Several quick responses are available for this one:
You: "Is the eat-or-be-eaten model the one we want to adopt and encourage?"
You: "Do you know what percentage of animals are carnivorous?"
You: "Humans spend most of their time denying their connections to animals, until they want to justify eating animals."

They: "Well, plants have life, too."
You: "If you are really concerned about that, you should become a vegetarian. Meat eaters are responsible for the deaths of all the plants that animals eat and then eat the animals, too."

They: "But what will happen to all the animals?"
You: "Do you assume vegetarianism will take over that quickly?"

They: "Do you eat fish or chicken?"
You: "Do fish or chicken grow from seeds?"
Or
You: "Do fish or chicken grow on trees?"

They: "Why are you wearing leather?"
You: "Let me see: does this question mean that if you are eating chicken and see a man beating a dog, you should not save the dog?"★

★Advocates for animals should probably adopt a consistent ethic, and it's wise to avoid wearing animal products if you aren't going to eat them for ethical reasons. If one "must" wear leather, then perhaps you could say, "I'm trying to reduce harm to animals, and perhaps I shouldn't have leather shoes. But we must all make choices, and hopefully our choices reflect our core values. Let me share with you some good literature on vegetarianism, and after you look at it perhaps we can talk about ways we might *both* reduce harming animals."

They: "Being a vegetarian must be hard."
You: "It was harder for me to live with the awareness that I was
  a meat eater."

They: "It's not practical."
You (shrugging your shoulders casually, in a light, dismissive
  manner to the concern): "It is."

When someone takes your vegetarianism personally:
You: "Why do you feel this is about you?"

They: "It's too much trouble."
You: "So's heart bypass surgery."

THE NATURE OF QUESTIONS

Questions reveal a great deal, more than most of us realize. *Listen to their questions, not to answer them, but as explanations.*

Some Questions Reveal How the Meat Eater Got Blocked

One of my children's friends came to our house when he was four. He was very upset. During a meal at McDonald's, he had announced to his parents that he wanted to be a vegetarian like my son. They told him he could not have his dessert unless he ate his Chicken McNuggets. He ate his meal and was rewarded with the dessert. Where did that vegetarian impulse go? It was buried in his psyche. He became a blocked vegetarian.

Three specific areas of concern often trace themselves backward to the questioner's childhood. These comments from meat eaters often announce how they got blocked:

- Declarations about suffering. "Animals don't suffer." Or "Animals don't have consciousness about suffering."

- Assumptions about existence. "This is why animals exist." "They would not exist if we didn't eat them." "At least they get to exist because they are going to be meat."
- Concern about needing meat to survive. And also simply to enjoy. "Why should I give up something I enjoy?"

Think about it: Where did your conversational partner develop this perspective? At a young age, those of us raised as meat eaters became conscious—at some point—that we were eating animals. What did we do with this information? In many cases we asked our parents or another authority figure. Unless they were extremely open meat eaters, they would explain that, yes, meat comes from dead animals, but one need not worry about that. Why not? They would most likely have answered us by saying:

- We need meat to survive.
- The animals would not exist unless we ate them *or* the animals exist so that we can eat them.
- They do not suffer.

Your parents may not have understood this themselves, but each of those answers is a lie. We do not need meat to survive. Vegetarians are proof of that. Animals *do* suffer. And animals can exist without our requiring them to be of service to us.

Whatever their age when children ask their parents or guardians about the meat on their plate—"Wasn't this an animal?"—from that point on, the concerns that motivated that question (concerns about why we have to eat animals) must go underground in the child's psyche. (Unless the parents allow the child's viewpoint to prevail and accept the child's vegetarianism.)

When, as an adult, a blocked vegetarian encounters a vegetarian, we stand there disproving what we all were told as children. We reveal to an adult that they were lied to at a very early age. This process of revelation might be happening below the surface of consciousness. When they throw these unfounded assumptions at us, and we respond, we aren't really arguing with the meat eater, but with those beliefs that were enforced at a very young age. And in arguing with those beliefs, we are very, very threatening!

The primal nature of these questions explains why, no matter what the setting, these questions in one form or another are raised. When I have spoken in scholarly settings, I have been surprised to hear variations of these questions in defense of meat eating! The concerns of the academics were no more sophisticated than the concerns of the non-scholarly meat eater. They held to the same concerns because these are the beliefs they had to accept, at a young age, in order to be obedient. The result? They became blocked.

Another early childhood experience influences the viewpoint of meat eaters. As very young children we think that when our parents or other caretakers cannot be seen, they have disappeared. We have a magical view of the world. When we hear that animals exist for our use, it fits in to this magical and decidedly egocentric view—the world exists for *us*. Though the magical view and the egocentric view may be challenged in other areas of a person's life, this particular belief is reinforced by the larger society. Vegetarians and animal rights activists immediately threaten this viewpoint by saying it is not true; animals do not exist for us. The way a child—albeit a now-grown child—made sense of their world is threatened.

Questions About Hitler Tell You Immediately That You Are Talking with a Very Defensive Meat Eater

Expect to get questions about Hitler's vegetarianism. Not *whether* Hitler was a vegetarian, but *how do you explain it?* The idea that Hitler *was* a vegetarian is a meat eater's security blanket. Remove it with great caution. Contained within the question is a justification: "Just because you are a vegetarian doesn't make you a better person, because you can be a vegetarian and be very bad. Just look at Hitler. So you aren't better than I am." The unspoken presumption in this question is "So who do you think you are, Mr. Holier-Than-Thou?"

Now, if you wish, you can get pulled into a debate about this. One way is to examine the facts in the case. After all, Hitler's "vegetarianism" was actually part of a Nazi public relations campaign to portray him as ascetic and "pure." You could try to say, "Many people don't know that Hitler was actually not a vegetarian and that this was just Nazi propaganda. In fact, vegetarian societies were proclaimed illegal when Hitler came to power. But is Hitler's diet important today? It seems to me, the real question you are struggling with is whether we, today, should be vegetarian. If you would like to receive some information, I'd be glad to send you some literature. . . ."

You could respond by trying to suggest that using the idea that Hitler was a vegetarian to tarnish all of vegetarianism is slightly illogical. After all, Hitler was against smoking, too, and implemented antismoking policies. Does this mean that antismoking activism today is tainted by Hitler's position? Of course not.

You can simply say, "So what?" After the meat eater explains why this matters to them, it could be pursued further . . . so what? And so what? again. However, you won't be seen as very friendly.

The real question is "What does the idea of Hitler's vegetarianism say to the meat eater?" It is functioning as a blocking device. People want to see themselves as moral. They may be thinking, "Just because Hitler was a vegetarian didn't make him a better person, so *not* being a vegetarian doesn't make me any less moral, because I am certainly a better person than Hitler."

You might also want simply to copy this section and carry it around. I have found that most people who use the "Hitler was a vegetarian" argument are pleased with themselves for knowing this supposedly historical information. They see themselves as offering a unique—and unanswererable—argument. When shown that this issue is actually anticipated, and is also quite frequent for vegetarians, this in itself might take the wind out of their sails.

In response to claims that are more complex and cannot be refuted so cleanly, we might say, "That's a complex issue, but I think you'd have to agree that being vegetarian does help reduce [hunger/animal suffering/environmental degradation/etc.]." This method does not presume that every question must be answered. It does not accept the unspoken agenda of the meat eater (to keep you on the defensive). When you hear a question, ask yourself: "Do I really need to answer this question?"

There Are Many Ways to Answer the Question "Why Are You a Vegetarian?" Choose the Most Effective One

First of all, remember that you do not have to answer this question, even though it may be the most tempting one to answer. But it creates as many problems as it solves. Of course, meat eaters don't really know what they are asking. They do not anticipate that the answer is going to speak to their current eating habits. What will the meat eater read into the answer? And do we wish to make ourselves vulnerable? Telling our vegetarian story can make us vulnerable because we are sharing something pivotal in our lives. Whom do we trust with this story? Here are several ways to answer the "why" question without accepting it as the agenda:

> "I don't think I will answer that. Let's just leave it that I'm a vegetarian. I am happy with the decision and happy to talk about it with you, but let's discuss it later."

> "Just because. I'm not trying to be difficult or evasive, but it's just because it felt right. I can't be more precise than that."

> "I'll tell you why I decided to become a vegetarian, if you will tell me why you choose to continue to be a meat eater."

If you decide to answer the question by actually describing the process by which you became a vegetarian, be prepared. Know yourself. Here is a simple self-assessment to complete. Take a moment and finish this sentence: "I am a vegetarian because . . ." Write down your answer, being as complete as possible. The purpose of this exercise is to clarify your own position while identifying your "hot buttons." The reasons you became a vegetarian are your hot buttons. If you became a vegetarian for health reasons, people will attribute every sniffle, cough, or flu to your vegetarianism. If it was for ethical reasons, people will unknowingly and knowingly trample on your ethics simply by being a part of your life. Should your reason be the environment, can people connect to your view of vegetarianism as an environmental issue? When you are done writing as expansively as possible, compress your answer into one clear sentence.

At times, a discussion can be open, engaging, supportive. A vegetarian can feel affirmed through telling his or her story, and an unthreatened meat eater can feel enlightened. I know that this is possible, I just don't assume it is frequent. But here's an example of a successful telling of the story of one's vegetarianism:

> Last summer, at the age of twenty-five, I contracted chicken pox. I was itchy and feverish during a heat wave in the high 90s. I was stuck in an apartment without air-conditioning, and was utterly miserable.
>
> I went to the local clinic and was given a prescription for antihistamines to bring to the pharmacy. The pharmacist gave me a bottle of capsules, which I looked at glumly. "Do you have any pills?" I asked, knowing that there's lactose in the pills as a filler, but trying to minimize the ickiness. After speaking a moment or two, I was able to exchange the cow-foot capsules for a large bottle of children's liquid. Yech. Anyway, the pharmacist and I engaged in a long discussion about why I was vegan and under what circumstances I would use animal products. He was very interested and asked polite questions, which I answered in a nonpreachy way.

When it was time to go, he asked if he could get anything else for me. Jokingly, I said I'd like a straitjacket to keep myself from scratching. With a totally straight face, he said, "I'd love to help you, but all of our straitjackets are made of leather." I just about died laughing.

This was his way of telling her, "I heard you."

CONVERSATIONS AMONG EQUALS

Two types of conversations among equals are my concern. The first is when you can help a meat eater to feel welcome and accepted, thus enabling him to explore what it is that keeps him blocked. This is very tricky and must be accomplished very carefully. Attack will quickly follow if you fail to keep the conversation on a nonjudgmental level. The other type of conversation is one between vegetarian equals. To discuss specific aspects of vegetarianism, there must be an even playing field. Your bottom line should be, "The meat eater shall not be allowed to be more familiar with me than circumstances allow." We'll turn to that one first.

Artificial Familiarity

"What about plants?" In asking you about the suffering of plants, meat eaters imply that a basic commitment to reducing harm is shared. But in actuality it isn't. With another vegetarian, I might explore my feelings about this sense of a plant's life. But not with a meat eater. I am giving them power over me. There is no equality of concern. In becoming a vegetarian, I have already made steps to stop suffering. They do not share my commitment; they have not made those steps. Since meat eaters who bring up these issues are not at the same level of engagement with the issues of suffering as the vegetarian is, we cannot engage with them as equally familiar with the issues as we are.

111

When a meat eater responds, "Well, what about plants?" you can say, "I've decided to do the least harm possible." And turn the question back to them: "What's your ethical bottom line?"

"What Are You Going Through?": Hearing the Meat Eater's Story

More important than conversation may be listening. Meat eaters are struggling with something you have resolved. They may be scared. Enact compassion for the nonvegetarian. They might not even understand that they are struggling with the issue. To their conscious mind, everything is all right. But the behavior you are now able to discern tells you otherwise. They have a need to hear you as well as a need not to hear you, and these needs are in conflict. In hearing would come the knowledge that change is possible. They would then have to recognize that they have to act. But then they would realize that something internal is keeping them from acting. Until they understand why they resist acting, their interaction with you will be fraught with implicit and explicit attacks against you.

On the other hand, we have no need *not* to hear. If they argue on behalf of meat eating, we've certainly heard that before. It isn't going to cause us to desert what we are doing. We cannot always help them learn how to hear us, but in listening to them we can show them how one listens. We can hear the meat eater's story.

One vegetarian reported to me, "People say things like, 'Oh—I guess my eating this chicken leg must look really disgusting to you. I hope I'm not grossing you out.'" This statement reveals that the meat eater is growing in consciousness—they have realized that a chicken leg can look disgusting to someone. They haven't internalized this feeling, but they intuit that it exists. The vegetarian who told me of this interaction paused and said, "I never have the nerve to say, 'Yes, you are [grossing me out].' *Should* I?" In a sense, the chicken eater has already realized what he or she is doing. The vegetarian could help this blocked individual more by responding, "Now that you are aware of what you are doing, how does it look to you?"

You can say to a meat eater, "The question is, When you look at meat what do you see? Not, What do *I* see?" Then you could ask, calmly, sincerely, "What do you do with the knowledge that you are eating dead animals?"

My feeling is that people who eat meat have deadened a part of themselves. They have been taught to deaden that part that cares about themselves, their health, the animals, the environment. Is this fair? I don't know. I know this is how I survive. My question then becomes not "How do I answer their questions about meat eating and vegetarianism?" but, in a very symbolic way, "How do we raise the dead?"

Our role is to get out of the way of the meat eater's process, not to be the target for their feelings. You can listen to clues other people give you about themselves. If someone says, "I cannot handle anything else! I can't handle any more changes!" we need to be able to hear them and ask, "What are you going through?"

You could continue with a question such as "Did you have a pet when you were a child?" Asking them to remember how they felt about that relationship allows them to touch that part of themselves that was alive to the lives of animals. Ask questions that signal empathy, not "message." "How did that feel? What are you going through?" Empathy teaches meat eaters how to ask and how to hear what another is going through.

The meat eater's story is actually more important than the vegetarian's story. The meat eater needs to deal with the past—that is what is keeping them locked to this way of life.

When someone says, "I tried vegetarianism for a while, but it was too hard" sometimes I respond by saying, "Tell me about it. What was hard exactly? Think back." Whatever triggers the response "hard" is where the energy got blocked. Maybe the answer is "Eating out with others." Well, then, they could strategize alternative ways of eating out. Or you can offer an empathetic, supportive statement like, "We all try to minimize harm to others. I'd be glad to help you try to reduce or eliminate meat from your diet. Perhaps this time it won't feel hard."* People who have tried to be vegetarians don't realize they just tried the wrong way. They haven't found the right way yet. Perhaps in talking to us they might discover this. But don't count on it. Be prepared to stop any conversation.

---

* *The Inner Art of Vegetarianism Workbook* offers a very gentle way of becoming vegan. I wrote it with blocked vegetarians in mind.

7

Stopping the Conversation

What is often a first encounter for a meat eater—talking to a vegetarian—is rarely a first encounter for that vegetarian. In most cases, we have been talking to meat eaters all our lives. Sometimes we need to stop talking. And in order to stop talking, we need to know how to stop the conversation.

"Why does everyone want to know why I am vegan?" a young woman asked me plaintively. "I'd like to gather them all around and tell them all at once. Give them a lecture on veganism, and be done with it. Instead, every time I eat with them I have to explain it over and over again." She lifted her hands in a gesture of helplessness. I told her, "The meat eater often sets the agenda. Curious or hostile, friendly or irritated, it doesn't matter. They may simply be looking for entertainment. Are you going to oblige them?" I reminded her, "This is hard work, answering everyone's questions. It keeps them occupied, and keeps you from enjoying your meal. They want to control the conversation, and you. You don't have to accept their agenda."

I learned this advice the hard way. I used to be like her.

When I lived in upstate New York, a friend visiting from Manhattan and I were invited to a dinner. Everyone there, except us, was associated with the local university; most were professors. One English professor in specific leaped into a defense of meat eating the minute he learned I was a vegetarian. I argued passionately answering each of his arguments with a counterargument. As we left the dinner, my friend said, "Do you go through that every time you eat with meat eaters?" Only then did I realize that yes, I did go through that all the time. Once I recognized this pattern of defending vegetarianism, I also realized how draining it was to engage in debate that way. I recaptured that experience in *The Sexual Politics of Meat*, when I discuss what happens with conversations. I wrote that conversations where meat is present will have to defeat the vegetarian:

> *As though a text of meat must be recapitulated on the level of discourse—the flesh made word—you become the rabbit, the other person the hunter who must vindicate the sport. You will be teased, you will be baited. . . . Though you are kept under control by this control of conversation, you appear to be the manipulator, the one who is redefining, delimiting, disempowering meat eating, and the other is the protector of the meaning of meat eating. . . . At a dinner where meat is eaten, the vegetarian must lose control of the conversation. . . . In this situation, the issue of vegetarianism is a form of meat to meat eaters: it is something to be trapped and dismembered.*

As I wrote those words, that debate with the English professor was prominent in my mind. I could recall all of the arguments that I, taking the event literally, had tried to rebut. I was always alert and on my toes. I remembered being exhausted after the confrontation, and I could imagine the young woman in a similar situation. Indeed, I could imagine numerous vegetarians all over the country undergoing what the young woman and I endured.

I wish I had known then what I know now: *You have the right to stop a conversation.* It's as simple as that. When you feel a conversation getting out of control, when you feel tired, if you just want to eat your meal, if you feel picked on, or when meat eaters have started to become defensive—stop the conversation. You do not have to answer their questions, respond to the challenges. You can develop new instincts for conversations, a new threshold for what is acceptable, and a new independence in relating to meat eaters' questions and concerns. You do not have to be trapped by a conversation.

Conversations get endowed with such freight that we think they are the most important interaction between meat eaters and vegetarians. They are merely the most frequent. Stop the conversation and discover that another level of interaction is possible.

WHY WE SHOULD STOP CONVERSATIONS

We've all heard the saying "The map is not the territory." The problem with conversations is that they keep meat eaters looking at *their* map. Even worse, conversations often keep *us* looking at *their* map! And their map doesn't include *our* territory. This is why we need to stop the conversations.

As we have seen in the earlier chapters, talking may be a means of avoiding vegetarianism rather than what it seems to be at first, a way of engaging it. Meat eaters are hoping you will help them short-circuit their own thinking. The more you talk or argue with them, the less they have to follow their own thought processes. The maxim "The best defense is a good offense" proves itself over and over in meat eater–vegetarian conversations. We should stop the conversation when we realize that meat eaters have chosen this tactic.

Then there is the problem of stubbornness. Meat eaters may stick their feet into the ground, saying to themselves, "I am not going to budge from this position." Stubbornly holding one's ground is not engagement. It is avoidance.

Let us remind ourselves how these conversations actually unfold.

The meat eater says, "Yes, but what about . . ." and she draws upon an issue from the last chapter: "Hitler?"; "protein?"; "plants?"; etc.

We reply, earnestly: "Well, Hitler wasn't a vegetarian," or "The average vegetarian, like the average meat eater, consumes twice as much protein as they need in a day," or "You don't really think a cow and a plant are similar, do you?"

Then the meat eater persists, saying, "Yes, but what about . . ." and they either intensify the question they were asking ("Everything I've read says Hitler was a vegetarian") *or* they change to another issue ("What about plants, proteins, etc.?").

And we earnestly respond to *this* statement.

What the persistent, argumentative meat eater is really saying is, "I will not let you get near me!"

The meat eater is hastily erecting a picket fence to keep vegetarian consciousness out. When we answer each issue they throw at us in situations like this, letting them dart from question to question, we tell them, "This method you have chosen of placing pickets in front of your consciousness is okay with me." We help them hammer in rigidity, though we are not aware that this is what we are doing. We take their arguments literally. We should not.

The poet Yeats observed that the most important arguments are with yourself. This is true for meat eaters, too. We have to know how to get out of the way of meat eaters' inner processes and allow them the opportunity for inner reflection. This is another reason to stop the conversation.

Conversations that occur over a meal usually leave as many people out of the conversation as they include. You stop a conversation at this point because other people are feeling left out of the conversation and they are going to blame you, not the meat eater, for monopolizing the discussion. People want to feel included. When a conversation has been reduced to a one-on-one debate, they will not feel included. And if everyone *is* included in this conversation, you need to stop it because you are being ganged up on. It is perfectly all right to stop the conversation because you need it to stop. You get tired. You become defensive. You want to relax. So, you stop a conversation to defuse a situation; to make an uncomfortable situation less so; to take the pressure off you to answer any and all questions posed.

You stop a conversation, too, because *our* vegetarianism has created *their* identity as meat eaters. This creates a sense of separateness. We have to find ways of helping them acknowledge our commonalities, not our differences, ways in which they can identify with us, rather than enact hostilities toward us.

You stop the conversation because the part of the brain that processes emotions works slower than the part that uses words. At times when we are feeling uncomfortable we speed up in talking, and thus we don't let our emotions interact with our words.

You stop the conversation because meat eaters do not respond to vegetarianism solely on the conscious level. People need time to process information at a deeper level, one that does not require consciously interacting with it. This is a process of incubation. With incubation, the slower we move, the faster we learn. Vegetarians who allow for incubating time report that they frequently hear, "You know, I've been thinking about your reasons to avoid meat, and while I'm not going to become vegetarian, I didn't eat a hamburger yesterday. . . ." As one correspondent wrote, "From that step, I've had eight friends become vegetarian." They needed time to incubate the ideas. They needed to set their own pace.

The idea that meat eaters are incubating vegetarianism at a level deeper than the conscious one explains why saboteurs over time become vegetarians.

You stop the conversation because both of you are getting short-winded. In a heated conversation, you are probably taking shorter and shorter breaths. Short breaths create a feeling of panic, of losing control.

Finally, you should stop a conversation if there is a predator—or if you are becoming one.

THE PREDATOR IN CONVERSATIONS

Sometimes a conversant is prowling around your emotional and intellectual arguments looking for the weak spot, biding his time, waiting for the moment when he can leap, throttle you, and defeat you. He is a predator.

A predator feels the need to vindicate meat eating. To the predator, vindicating meat eating requires defeating you. Not only your message but you, sitting there with your vegetables and rice, must be thrown upon the floor and bloodied. The predator believes conversations should be battles, that there are victors in conversations. And if there are victors, there are also the vanquished. The predator, at all costs, cannot allow herself to be defeated. She will slay the enemy—metaphorically speaking, doing to the vegetarian what the slaughterer did to the animal.

You become the prey by announcing that you are a vegetarian. It is much safer, always, not to have an opinion and not to be identified as different. A vegetarian who is "discovered" or self-proclaimed does not have that choice. She has been identified. Whereas other people might speak in generalities, and don't commit themselves, in making observations such as "It is always better to . . ." we have already given ourselves away. The predator will notice that. It is as though you are the weak or older or sick member of a group of zebras escaping a lion. You become the target for the lion.

Once there is a predator, either he wins or you win. Neither sight is pretty. If you fight with a predator, a "victory at all cost" meat eater already defensive in your presence may begin to think that you aren't listening to him, and your responses may be proving him right. If your goal is to push the confrontation, then it really becomes about you: you become "relentless"; "She just won't give up"; "He doesn't allow other perspectives."

It is very difficult for a vegetarian to "win" a conversation when meat is being eaten. Too much is at stake at that moment for meat eaters to relent at the verbal level. Indeed, everyone else may be secretly cheering the predator on.

You must throw the lion off the scent. To do this, you have to stop being so easily targeted. You have to stop the conversation.

TAKING THE PULSE OF A CONVERSATION

To determine if a conversation should be stopped, you need to know how to take the pulse of a conversation. Here are several questions to ask yourself to determine whether a conversation should continue:

- Are they eating meat?
- Are they hounding you? Trying to embarrass you? Can you tell by their behavior that they are busy marshaling their army of arguments rather than listening to your responses?
- Are you feeling angry, upset, impatient, teased, baited? The question is not What are you *saying,* but Have you fallen into the old pattern in which your mind has simply galloped forward in its habitual way to explain, defend, educate?
- Are they speaking loudly?
- Have all other conversations ended? Do people look annoyed or bored?
- Is shame happening? Are you shaming them or are they shaming you? (Examples of shaming language: "Everyone knows that you . . ." "Even you . . ." "You always . . .") Have you become the topic of the conversation or have you made them the issue?
- Are people interrupting each other? (If a meat eater is interrupted, everyone at the table will believe that you are not listening. They will feel more threatened because they will assume you have already judged them, and want to convert them, not hear them.)
- Is the body language hostile? Raised eyebrows? Knowing glances between meat eaters? Condescending smirks? Jabbing of fingers in the air or raising clenched fists?
- Is your heart racing or do you feel short of breath?

If the answers to any of these questions are yes, stop the conversation.

STOPPING THE CONVERSATION

It is your responsibility to stop a conversation. As we have seen, most meat eaters want conversations to continue as long as they can control them.

If you begin to discuss the issue, have in your mind a cut-off point: "If I hear [X question], I'll know . . ." or "If the pulse becomes . . . I'll know . . ."; "When I hear 'Yes, but . . .'" Review in your mind the nonverbal signs that will act as cues.

And then what should you do? One person advises, "Tell them to shut up and eat their carcass." I think there are gentler ways.

You may decide to be a broken record. If you are being confronted repeatedly by offers of meat it might be, "No thank you." If you are being interrogated about your reasons, select a one-liner (see pages 102–105) and simply repeat it.

Remember: show, don't tell. Get their snail-mail address, fax number, or e-mail address and offer to send them some information or Web site addresses. This lets them know that you hear their interest but do not accept their timeline. If they are truly interested, they will be thankful. If they are not truly interested, it will be obvious and then *you* can be thankful. You can say, "Let's not talk about that now, but I would be glad to give you some information. Give me your [e-mail address, fax number, etc.] and I'll send you some material."

Leapfrog to another subject. "Of course some people say that vegetarianism is only a part of a larger change. Have you noticed how many organic farmers there are?" Or, "Yes, I have seen that suggested on the Internet. By the way, do you think the Internet . . . [and ask some news-related question about the Internet]." Almost everyone has an opinion on this subject.

Make a joke.

Flatter the host, the chef, the person you are sitting next to.

Stop a conversation. Sometimes that is exactly what is needed. You will be remembered, gratefully, by most of your fellow diners for being gracious under pressure.

8

Love at Work I: Living with Meat Eaters

The Nature of Relationships and Kitchens

Living with a meat eater is no worse than living with a cat. My meat-eating husband is much more considerate than my cats: he does not expect me to buy his meat or prepare it and he NEVER, NEVER vomits on my place on the table as my cats regularly do.

— MARIA

iving with meat eaters—roommates, parents, family, and lovers—is living with divided loyalties. It demands a balancing act. You have probably heard the adage "Happy families are all alike; every unhappy family is unhappy in its own way." Tolstoy, a vegetarian, said that. This adage takes on a different edge when some of the unhappiness in a family or a relationship is caused by a conflict in food choices, or at times with what even qualifies as "food." Each meat-eating family's conflicts with a vegetarian family member follows similar patterns. The problem is, most people think that such family or relationship dramas are uniquely theirs.

Your conflicts will be of two kinds: those that arise with them because they are blocked or conflicts that arise with you because you aren't. You are being asked to love them in their blockedness more than they love you in your unblockedness. Sometimes this is hard, very hard.

How they relate to you is determined by what is blocking them. Sometimes in our relationships with them, we cause their well-developed defenses to erode. On the other hand, especially with partners, our vegetarianism may result in their becoming more strongly committed to meat eating.

Here is the problem: no matter how important your relationship with them is, most meat eaters are going to choose to continue to eat meat. They will change only when they are ready, not when you *need* for them to change. If you begin relationships with meat eaters, you have to understand this fact. If you are continuing relationships with meat eaters after becoming a vegetarian, you also have to understand this fact. No matter how important vegetarianism is to you, and no matter how important you are to a meat eater, these two compelling facts will not convert most meat eaters into vegetarians. Does this mean you are condemned to incompatibility? No. Incompatibility does not arise from differences. Incompatibility arises from whatever prompts these differences to stand out. The question is, How do you maintain a relationship with a meat eater who is going to continue to eat meat? And how do you share kitchen and dining space with conflicting diets?

CAREFULLY.

Be realistic. . . . But understand your limitations.

Be able to negotiate for your interests. . . . But understand where you can compromise.

RELATIONSHIP ISSUES

We want our loved ones to be happy. We want them to enjoy special meals, in both the anticipation of a meal and the eating of it. We know that there is a certain kind of happiness that occurs when one is eating a good meal. But for them special meals include meat. So we may experience a conflict between wanting a loved one or companion to be happy and watching them eat meat.

In interactions with meat eaters, you generally have to cultivate some sort of distancing. If it is physical distancing, this means you make a decision not to associate with meat eaters. Then you rarely have relationship issues. Most vegetarians are not able to draw this line in the sand. They have associations with meat eaters because of family, work, friendships, volunteering, or housing situations. If your vegetarianism is important to you, you may vacillate among three main feelings:

- Denial. You say to yourself, "They are okay people [for, of course, they really are], and I can ignore their food choices."
- Anger. "Why, if they are okay people, are they making the food choices they are making?" This also leads, sometimes, to self-righteousness: "Why aren't they listening to me, why aren't they respecting my opinion?" Our egos are hard at work with this one.
- Acceptance. "They are okay people and I can't change them. And we love each other despite this difference." Or, "They are okay people and they are also responsible for the deaths of animals and I can't change them. I have to live with the sorrow and that paradox."

Displaced Conflict

Any unresolved aspects of the relationship—unequal power such as that between parent and child, gender roles, old wounds never healed—will attach themselves to vegetarian–meat-eating dynamics. The tensions are caused by something else but they find expression in discussions and debates about food choices. Your vegetarianism and their meat eating become burdened with representing basic relationship issues—issues of control, especially. The debate might appear to be about what was eaten at supper, but it really is about something else.

Because food differences may bear the burden of basic relationship conflicts, meat eaters may use their meat eating to represent something else: it can be punishment, control, insecurity. They may be declaring independence from the vegetarian, who is seen as being the controlling one. If the meat eater views abstaining from meat at a meal as giving up a part of oneself, they may view eating a vegetarian meal as "giving in" to the vegetarian roommate/partner/family member. The power equilibrium will be thrown off and the meat eater will try to restore it through whatever means possible.

The Art of Disagreeing

- Be clear about the issue. Repeat it.
- Watch out for extraneous issues that complicate it, making it more difficult to respond. If the issue is the frying pan or cooking utensils or the cutting board, don't use it as a way to criticize his or her meat eating or for your vegetarianism to be criticized.
- Listen to the other. What is the other's point of view? You may disagree with it, but do you know it?
- Don't raise your voice during an argument.
- Don't fight to win.
- Don't say, "Why are you doing this?" or, "You're always . . ." accusingly, as though the partner/roommate/family members are deliberately doing something to "harm" you.
- Remember that during times of disagreement, no one is a reliable historian. So don't use the conflict to remind the other person of other "errors" of the past.

In negotiating and in disagreements, the person with the least at stake (or who cares the least about something) has the most power. In many negotiations involving relationship and household issues, you are going to care more about vegetarianism than the people you live with do. This often creates unequal power dynamics. The less invested, the easier it is to walk away from any negotiation.

SHARED KITCHENS

A friend of a friend of mine was sharing student accommodation with a bunch of in-your-face, obnoxious meat eaters. They used to go home to Mummy and Daddy on the weekend, leaving her alone in the flat. Incensed by their attitude, she started removing their meat from the freezer every weekend, defrosting it, and then putting it back before they returned. They all got food poisoning and she moved out.

—A VEGETARIAN URBAN MYTH

Well, this is one way to handle the challenge of sharing a kitchen with meat eaters. The problem for vegetarians is that *they* are more likely to get food poisoning from the contact of raw meat with cutting boards and knives than meat eaters are. Of all the dynamics of living with a meat eater, kitchen issues are the most practical. They often feel the most pressing as well. They aren't, they just feel that way.

The Top Kitchen Concerns of Vegetarians

- Should I share cutting boards? Their salmonella-laden chicken may contaminate the cutting board, and anything of yours that comes in contact with it. Your problem: their food will probably be cooked; you are more likely to eat your veggies and fruits raw. You therefore are more susceptible to salmonella poisoning.
- Should I share utensils and cookware with meat eaters or should I have dedicated cookware?
- Do I have to cook food with meat in it for others?

- Does the dishwasher really clean the plates and utensils, or will meat residue linger?
- Does my vegetarian food have to share refrigerator space with meat and dairy?
- Do I have to smell meat cooking?
- Do I have to shop for food nonvegetarians eat that I don't eat?

Prioritize Your Issues

What concerns you the most in sharing a kitchen? The smells? Reactions to the smell of meat cooking can be pretty intense. One correspondent told me:

I now feel physical sickness (mostly nausea and loss of appetite) when I smell cooked flesh. And seeing it makes me want to cry. It is hard for me in general to eat meals with meat eaters, but I am the only vegetarian in the family.

Another wrote:

Being around someone cooking steak was the most recent and disgusting. The smell was just rotten and all I could smell was dead animal and it just strengthened my resolve to continue being vegetarian. I left the room and wouldn't return until the smell had gone.

Or are you concerned about the chores and having a fair distribution that does not require you to interact with meat dishes? Who will clean dishes used to store, prepare, or serve meat?

Examine the kitchen concerns identified above and determine which ones need to be addressed: cutting board, shared cookware, chores, smells, shared refrigerator space. Is there some flexibility in the kitchen that can accommodate your needs? Are there other areas of household management that can be incorporated into a new arrangement?

Negotiating about kitchen concerns is like negotiating about other aspects of a relationship: know your bottom line and know where you can compromise. For instance, the issue of pots and pans. Solution: identify some pans and knives that will be used only to cook vegetarian food. When proposing this, describe the practical needs for it, and use a tone of voice that is even and nonjudgmental. It requires cooperation. Do you have it from your meat eater housemates?

This is what Maria worked out with her partner:

Although my avoidance of meat is based on ethical reasons, I do not want to be contaminated with it: his meat touching my food has become a symbol of unwilling participation in a massacre. For this reason, it is surprising to see how scrupulous (even more scrupulous than myself) he is. He uses his own pots and pans and utensils, he confines his meat to the enclosed area of the refrigerator.

Maria continues:

I do have one health concern: because my husband brings raw meat in the house, I, and not he, run the risk of food poisoning. This is because he always cooks everything, including all his vegetables, and I eat a lot of raw food. Washing the kitchen counter does not eliminate the risk. He does not pour boiling water or other disinfectant every time he cleans up, nor do I expect him to.

You need your household to understand this problem and you need their cooperation. Have your own cutting board that meat eaters promise they will not use. If you are sharing a cutting board, ensure that any cutting boards used to cut raw meat are washed with boiling water before you use them.

If you don't have cooperation in this cutting board problem, what does this tell you and what can you do about it? Is there something they need from you? Something else you can compromise on?

If you have "dedicated" knives, cutting boards, and pans and the meat eater(s) you are living with fail to respect their vegetarian nature—you have a practical problem, but you also have an even more serious problem. You are living with people who aren't respecting you. The relationship has changed in more ways than you thought.

IF YOU ARE THE PRIMARY COOK IN A HOUSEHOLD OF MEAT EATERS

You live with meat eaters, but you have become a vegetarian. You also share or have sole meal preparation responsibilities. What do you do? Negotiate new arrangements.

Do you wish to continue cooking meat? That is a primary issue. If you are comfortable doing so, there is nothing to negotiate. Many people who become vegetarians want to bring their partner, families, or household along with them. How can they do that?

Remember, incompatibility does not arise from differences; it arises from whatever prompts them to stand out. Your role is not so much to continue feeding them meat if you no longer wish to prepare it but to ease them through these new differences so that they don't stand out.

How do you do this? Negotiate. Explain what you can and can't do and offer alternatives. If you have children, you may want to explain to them, depending on their ages, why you have decided to become a vegetarian. Be clear what your expectations for your children are. You can say, "This is what I can no longer do. I can't fix hamburger, chicken, or turkey anymore." But: "You can fix it." Or:

"I will fix ethnic food (pasta, stir-fry, burritos), and you can fix the meat that could accompany that dish."

"There can be a meat eaters' night when you order in and I'll use that night to go out to eat at my favorite vegetarian spot/go with friends to a vegetarian potluck/attend a seminar on vegetarianism/[etc.]"

"I will learn how to prepare foods that make you not miss the meat." Food items such as texturized vegetable protein,* seitan, tofu dogs, and veggie burgers could become prominent in your list.

Read the section in Chapter 13 on eating the menu, not the meal, and remind yourself not to discuss the nature of the food you prepared as they eat it. They do not need to be consciously reminded of what they may feel they are missing. Afterward, you can ask for evaluations, or, as the case might be, if a meal elicits negative reactions, you'll know of their rejection pretty quickly. You can also have available as a backup a family standard (spaghetti, baked potato, etc.) and unhappy eaters can choose that option instead. Remind yourself that a family can handle change.

It is okay for *roles* to change as well as *diets*. As with any relationship issue, you need to know your bottom line (Let's say it is "I no longer wish to eat or prepare meat"), and understand where to compromise. Cook with a spirit of invitation: inviting them to you and negotiating about the needs they have that your vegetarian cooking can't meet.

Reeducating their palate can take a while—some estimate it takes about four months. Resistance makes it take longer. Perhaps they never accept your diet completely. It doesn't matter. Create alternative arrangements that share cooking responsibilities. Moving a family toward including more vegetarian items in their menus is a gift to their health. Helping them accept change in their diets or their roles teaches them how to become more open. Experiencing the art of negotiation around each one's needs shows them how to compromise lovingly.

---

*Texturized vegetable protein (TVP) is made from soy flour. According to Dorothy R. Bates, author of *The TVP® Cookbook: Using the Quick Cooking Meat Substitute* (Summerton, Tenn.: Book Publishing Co., 1991), p. 4: "TVP® is produced from soy flour after the soybean oil has been extracted, then cooked under pressure, extruded, and dried." From this process, a dense texture that is chewy and "meatlike" is produced. It is sold in granules, flakes, chunks, or slices. When rehydrated the granules resemble ground "beef" and the chunks have the texture and appearance of chunks of "meat." Especially, when cooked in certain ways, it is often mistaken for meat and it can be substituted for meat, such as "hamburger," in recipes like "sloppy joes." TVP® is an excellent source of protein and fiber, and has zero cholesterol. The initials are the registered trademark of the Archer Daniels Midland Company.

Involving them in kitchen responsibilities gives them each the gift of independence and the ability to express love through food preparation.

Handle conflict with the awareness of change and the potential of change. Then vegetarianism is a gift that keeps on giving.

9

Love at Work II: Living with Meat Eaters

The Family System

When one lives with another person or other people, a system evolves. It has to. Arrangements must be made for the mundane aspects of life such as cleaning the toilet and shopping, paying bills and fixing food. When we are children the system serves us. It directs us toward maturity by having rules and boundaries, and, when it works, it ensures that we are fed and rested. At some point, we acquire tasks in the system, gradually assuming a more active role in making decisions about our own lives. When we are teenagers the balancing act of being taken care of and participating in decision making tilts toward the latter or is pushed there by our needs to separate from the system.

A system needs rules and roles. Through rules and roles, the system achieves stasis, balance—it runs smoothly. Any change in one part of the system will provoke a change in another part. Because of this, huge changes don't have to occur to change the whole system. No matter its size, any real, substantive change, especially ones that arise from a sense of living a life of authenticity and integrity, can change the whole system.

There are in fact two kinds of change:

A first-order change shifts the playing pieces on the board, but the rules remain the same. For instance, one grows up. We are no longer "pawns" on a chessboard, but become the knight, or the bishop, or the rook. This is a first-order change.

A second-order change changes the rules of the game; chess is no longer played in the same way. You may see your desire to become a vegetarian as a simple change, say, from being a pawn to being a rook. Other members of your system experience your becoming a vegetarian as a second-order change. You are changing the rules of the game. Specifically, you are rejecting a basic rule of the house. "This is what we eat." "This is what a holiday meal is." "This is how we honor our ancestors, our culture, our parents." You can tell it is a second-order change because of the responses you receive, which often refer to fundamental ways of organizing the world.

In specific, four responses confirm that you are threatening a core aspect of the family system.

- "Why shouldn't I prepare food the way I want to?" The person who is the cook wishes his or her will to be respected. She or he sees you as not respecting that will.
- "This is how I do it." Convenience and custom are compelling aspects of any system. "I do it this way because it works."
- "My way is right." A refusal to be influenced by another, stubbornness, and conviction, especially if the cook is one of the people who shaped the system to begin with.
- "This is how I know you love me. You eat the food I prepare." Family systems are often organized around very perverse ways of expressing and needing love.

You need to understand this very clearly: *the system does not want to change.* No matter how hard it was for us to change, the system itself has even greater resistance. We have to hold to our standards, understanding that it is the job of the system not to change, and that it will try to bring us back into its old patterns.

No matter how much you believe that being a vegetarian in a meat-eating family can work, most meat-eating families, especially those where you are a child (even an adult child), do not believe it can work. And remember that the system has already handled this issue once. When? When, as a child, you raised the issue "Where does hamburger/chicken/pork chops come from?" The system at that point had several effective methods for responding and preserving itself:

- Authority: As we saw in Chapter 6, the parents can say, "Eat your Chicken McNuggets or you can't have dessert."
- A claim to greater knowledge: "This cow did not suffer."
- A sacrificial interpretation: "Cows exist to be eaten."
- A nutritional imperative: "You need to eat meat to survive."

These methods worked once: they caused you to become a blocked vegetarian. Why shouldn't they work again? You are the only one who will demonstrate that they don't work. But it isn't easy.

The system will recognize that you are older now, and will have to bring greater force to defeating you. Something will seem drastically urgent, demanding that you return to the person you were. Something will challenge the second-order change. This is resistance at work. It will be very powerful in its efforts to bring you back into the system. It doesn't want the rules to change. Indeed, the system will intensify around this issue for a while. You will be told how important it is that you conform to the family system—someone's feelings are at stake, or family tradition is being threatened, you are rejecting someone or something. If this attempt to bring you back into the system isn't working, efforts will be made to destroy you. Not literally, but to remove all the support that could be brought to maintain the person you are and instead get you to return to the person you were. This pressure feels almost unbearable.

So, what are you to do?

You wait it out. It will pass. The system can adjust; it can evolve to accept your vegetarianism. But before it does, you may feel a great deal of anguish. This is why you need to identify a bottom line regarding your vegetarianism, and know how to maintain it. That will protect you from the demands of the system.

IDENTIFYING YOUR BOTTOM LINE

In becoming a vegetarian, you discover what is acceptable to you and what is not. This is your bottom line. Your bottom line is what differentiates you from the system that does not want to change. You recognize and act on your bottom line because you understand that your duties to your family and friends are not unconditional. You can set limits. You say to yourself, "This is what I will no longer do. I will no longer participate in Thanksgiving dinner as we have known it. But this is what I will do: I will come (or I will arrive after the main course is over), I will fix a tofu turkey (or I will bring a great pumpkin pie). I will participate in the holiday in a new way." And once you clarify for yourself what it is that you can and cannot do, you are able to tell your family, too.

Take a moment now and identify your bottom line.

Are you willing to watch others eat meat? If no, arrange to eat separately.

Are you willing to bring or prepare several dishes or a dessert?

Are you willing to host the event and create a new tradition?

Your bottom line about vegetarianism is the place where you differentiate yourself from your family.

In order to establish a bottom line it will be critical to communicate a few things to your family. Such communication might consist of these points: 1) You very much appreciate efforts to prepare nutritious, tasty meals for you, but 2) You feel strongly about diet and you expect your choices to be respected, however much others disagree with you. Of course, you will continue to respect their dietary choices as well.

Do not confuse establishing and maintaining a bottom line with lecturing your family about it. The purpose of the bottom line is simply to protect your decision. Its purpose is not to interpret it or enforce it against others. Yes, you can talk about your decisions that led to this new and threatening bottom line, but follow the rules for talking with meat eaters (see Chapter 6). Remember, the consequences for your family of being blocked don't disappear simply because you are among them. In fact, as you understand by now, you make their being blocked more painful. They may want you to change and be the person you once were. This is resistance.

IDENTIFYING RESISTANCE AT WORK

Remember, incompatibility does not arise from differences; it arises from whatever prompts these differences to stand out.

The system prompts the differences to stand out because vegetarianism means change and consequently a challenge. Our families teach us how to respond to change. Granted, many of the responses we learned are self-defeating. From them we may have learned to respond defensively and with spite. We may have been fortunate and learned how to respond with openness and flexibility. Most of us, however, learned the well-developed self-defeating responses that keep the family system intact. It may be comforting, at some level, to understand that the family will continue to act in its traditional way. You can be prepared. You will have to lead the way in showing that differences do not mean incompatibility.

Intensification is the pressure, the emotional leverage, that will be brought against you for making your bottom line explicit to your family. And because you understand your bottom line, you can withstand this intensification. It might be experienced as imploring ("Just this one time"; "But it's Aunt Edna's family casserole!"), even begging ("Eat this for me!") or as the enforcement of rules through anger ("How dare you not eat this!"). With your bottom line in place you are able to resist the intensification around the issue. You wait it out. It may be a long wait. As my friend James reported to me, "I have been a vegetarian for eighteen years and it was only recently that my mother stopped cooking meat for me when I came home to visit her."

No matter. Like James, you say, "No thanks. I prefer to eat this instead."

You hold to your bottom line despite the system not changing. You will probably feel a variety of emotions prompted by the way the family system handles your vegetarianism. These feelings may include disappointment, isolation, rejection, depression from your family's lack of care about your situation. You need to tell yourself that this is a part of the system bumping up against your change. During this time you need to be sure that you are taking care of yourself. Remember, self-care is part of being at peace with your vegetarianism (see pages 26–27).

RESISTANCE TACTICS

You can predict that the resistance will happen. It may involve disguising meat in the hopes that you will eat it. Alarmed for you about your vegetarianism, a family member may slip meat or dairy into your meals without telling you. This is a desperate move on their part, but what it means is that they are choosing to violate your trust rather than let go of their beliefs in the traditional meals of the family and our culture.

I have told the story about the vegetarian whose mother fixed eggs in bacon grease and stopped pressing her to eat meat when her daughter got sick. The mother had to learn how to expand her sense of what caring/mothering involved. For her it had been associated with feeding children meat. She had to renegotiate her own self-definition to let go of the need to feed a child/young adult meat. She had to learn to be flexible.

What should you do? The minute you suspect someone is feeding you meat, you need to get more involved in the family's food preparation. Minimally, you could sit in the kitchen and keep the cook company or, more appropriately, begin to study recipe books and selecting foods that you are interested in preparing. If there is a way to do it without recycling blame and guilt, you could talk about how important it is to you to feel that you can trust your family members while also giving family members the benefit of the doubt. You can say, "You meant well," but explain that their actions caused you to feel hurt, because it violated your trust in them. Make clear that trust is critical to a loving relationship, and ask them to promise not to do this again.

VERBAL TACTICS

More frequent than disguising meat and tricking or misleading the vegetarian into eating it are verbal attempts to get a vegetarian to eat meat. Two favorite verbal tactics are shame and guilt. If you can strip them of their most potent weapons—surprise and accusation—resistance tactics are fairly unremarkable. If you aren't prepared for accusations, however, they can do a lot of damage. The first one is:

"If you *really* loved . . .

> me
> your grandmother
> your parents

> you would . . .

> eat meat."
> stop being a vegetarian."
> raise your kids as meat eaters."
> eat what your grandmother fixed for you."
> fix meat for me."

How strongly the word *really* is stressed will alert you to the strength of the resistance attempt. The presupposition here is that "you don't really love me." Your vegetarianism is actually incidental to this assumption and thus the interaction. It is taken simply as the most recent confirmation of a "given" within the system. Whatever makes you different (or disobedient) reveals your lack of love. It thus makes you vulnerable to an attack. For vegetarians, the difference is their vegetarianism.

What should you do? Don't respond to what the clause focuses on, the "you would eat meat [or whatever]." Don't get defensive as though you have been accused. This is one way you are showing you accept the system's dysfunctionality. Don't let them hook you to their blaming style. One way you communicate your nondefensiveness is by remaining detached. Avoid responding such as:

> *Loved one: "If you really loved me, you would eat meat."*
> *You: "Of course I love you. My being a vegetarian does not mean I don't love you."*

The problem with this response is that there is no need to defend yourself, and when there is no need to defend yourself, you should avoid sentences with "I" or "me." That keeps the focus on you and allows the loved one to win: their premise has been accepted. Love *is* expressed through eating the foods they prepare, and you *don't* love them. The system survives.

Also avoid accepting their premise and volleying it back to them:

> *Loved one: "If you really loved me, you would stop eating meat."*
> *You: "Well, if you loved me, you would start cooking more vegetarian meals/become a vegan/watch this video on meat production with me/[etc.]."*

The problem with this is that you accept the premise of the family system and simply reverse it. Blame is still going on. It's just that this time *you* make *them* defensive. This keeps any real dialogue from happening.

A way exists to affirm your relationship, reassure the other member of the family system that you are not destroying it, and remove your vegetarianism from the equation.

Loved one: "If you really *loved me, you would eat meat."*
You: "When did you start thinking I don't love you?"

This neutral response reassures them. Your loved one assumed something about your vegetarianism because this is what the family system said about how family members show love—by following family customs, by eating what is prepared for them, by eating meat. Your response indicates they were wrong in a gentle, affirmative way. The important thing is not letting the focus become your behavior. It is their assumptions that must be changed, not your behavior.

Another way to respond is:

Loved one: "If you really *loved me, you would eat meat."*
You: "You know, it's interesting that loved ones have this feeling that they are not loved if people in their family become vegetarians/vegans. This is a normal reaction, yet even though it has happened in other families, it is still interesting. Does the fact that I don't share your love of opera indicate that I don't love you? Does the fact that you don't share my love of baseball indicate that you don't love me?"

This response does not blame them back. It acknowledges that you have heard them, but it also acknowledges that this is not an area where you feel defensive. You are not going to get dragged into an argument or the ongoing cycle of blame and shame.

If blame doesn't work, how about guilt?

Loved one:
"Don't you even care that . . .   *. . . I did all the cooking?"*
                                      . . . I fixed your favorite food?"
                                      . . . everyone will be here?"
                                      . . . it's Thanksgiving/my birthday?"

. . . it would mean so much to me?"

. . . [anything else that is important to the speaker].

Now, in analyzing this interaction, I am presuming that the speaker knew you were a vegetarian, and had been told what you do and don't eat. If he spent a lot of time cooking a meal for you without knowing that you did not eat the foods prepared, you have neglected a basic aspect of relationships: communication. You also reveal that you don't care that he did all that cooking. You *should* feel guilty!

If you did remind someone that you were a vegetarian, and she is pressuring you to eat meat because of her cooking issues, you do not need to feel guilty, even though she wants you to. Remember, there is a lot of guilt floating around the issue of meat eating anyway. It is safer for nonvegetarians to have you feel guilty for changing than for them to feel guilty for not changing. Let's look at the presumptions in these guilt-bestowing statements.

"Don't you care that I did all the cooking?"
"You *don't* care that I did all the cooking."
"You *should* care that I did all the cooking."
"You are rotten not to care that I did all the cooking."
"Therefore you should feel guilty about this."

Your need at this time is to keep the system from intensifying the issue. The system has chosen guilt ("shouldas") in an attempt to make it unbearable for you to remain a vegetarian. For those in the system, guilt is a very handy tool. It keeps them in line. Why shouldn't it work the same on you? How do you respond? Ignore this defensive move. Don't get hooked.

The biggest impediment to being able to ignore the system's resistance is when you are a "scanner." A scanner is attuned to the other's emotional states, and believes it is her responsibility to take care of the other person's emotions. She believes, "I need to eat what my family/partner is eating, otherwise I will hurt their feelings." No, you don't need to. You are not responsible for how they interpret your self-differentiation. You are not responsible for taking care of their emotions. You are not only keeping them blocked, you will ensure that you become blocked again.

Instead, you can respond like this:

Loved one: "Don't you even care I cooked this for you?
You: "When did you start thinking that I didn't care?"
Loved one: "When you became a vegetarian."

You have two choices here:

1) You: "Do you know why I became a vegetarian?"

If your loved one says, "To upset me," you could say, "No. Not at all. I have some literature that provides information on vegetarianism. I became a vegetarian for the reasons this [book, pamphlet, article] discusses. I would be happy for you to look at it if it would help you understand my decision."

2) You: "You are the one who taught me to care and I have extended this sense of caring to other animals and the environment. Thank you for teaching me this!"

Loved one: "Don't you even care that it's Thanksgiving?"
You: "I love the [bean casserole, etc.] and I love sharing Thanksgiving with the family."
Loved one: "Well, why can't you eat the turkey then?"
You: "Because I have changed."

You can add, if you are speaking to a parent or grandparent, "You raised us to be compassionate and caring, and I have found an important focus for this."

There might be tears. "I never get to fix you your favorite gravy anymore." You listen. You, without getting defensive, say, "Thank you for letting me know about this. I am sorry it has been difficult for you.

It means so much to me that you want to cook my favorite foods. My favorite foods now are [and tell the cook what they are]."

Loved one: "If you really loved me you would eat what I prepared." The message here, needless to say, is "You don't love me. There is only one way you can show me that you indeed love me. That is to accept my standards for a meal."

When you hear the above statement or its corollary, "Don't you even care that I fixed this for you?" you are being told of the cook's disappointed expectations. "You don't love me, you don't eat the food I prepared." The cook equates rejection of food with rejection of themselves. The thing is not to feel guilty. This is not your responsibility, nor your fault. Any act that offers food and says more than "Let me share with you this good food" is an act of control. Cooking does not need to be about control, nor should it be.

You can say, "I love you, but I choose not to eat like you now. I prefer to eat something else. While I can't eat what you prepared, I appreciate your effort."

Or: "I'm very thankful for your efforts to prepare good meals for me. But you taught me to do what I believe is right, even if others disagree. How could I expect you to respect me if I did otherwise?"

One final volley of guilt remains:

Loved one: "If you really loved me, you wouldn't want to be a vegetarian."

Here you are really trapped. What can you do? Even if you ate the meal, you are already guilty of not *wanting* to eat it. You might have changed your actions to comply with their expectations, though it is doubtful that you will do so if you are happily vegetarian, but you cannot undo your already announced desires to eat differently. And you don't have to. In a healthy, functioning family, such signs of love would not be required.

Your reply: "My being a vegetarian is about me, not about you or how much I love you."

In Chapter 3, I provided a chart that distinguished between flow and control (page 41). The system wants control, not flow. That is what it teaches its members. The blood that runs in the veins of the system is anxiety. The challenge is to be self-differentiated (understanding and acting on your bottom line) and connected (a part of the family system without being controlled by it) at the same time. We do this simply by being at peace with our diet and refusing to be drawn into the dramas that anxiety causes as it snakes its way through the system: "No thank you. I don't want that. I love you and appreciate the [whatever they have cooked that you can eat]." We teach our families that we can reject the traditional family food and yet still love them.

Then the system will change. It may take a while, but the system will have to incorporate your bottom line into itself. One vegetarian told me, "My family says that I won't eat anything that has ever had an address." They are telling her, "We hear your concern. We accept your decision."

10

Love at Work III:
Living with Meat Eaters

Partners and Children

I n the best relationships, love is a complicated emotion. In a mixed (meat eater–vegetarian) relationship, our relationship gets even more entangled. This may be as easy to remedy as releasing a scarf caught in a door, but sometimes it causes the anxiety of a shoelace caught in the escalator treads.

Partner issues vary depending on when you became a vegetarian. If it is before you entered a committed relationship, your partner issues may be meeting a vegetarian. If you become a vegetarian after entering a committed relationship, your partner issues are loving a meat eater and perhaps also raising meat-eating children. Since this book addresses living among meat eaters, and since other avenues for addressing the issue of vegetarian singles exist (from on-line discussion groups to vegetarian singles groups in many urban areas), this section will concentrate on living *with* a meat eater.

DATING

"Carnivores are okay for one-night stands,
but for a relationship, give me a vegetarian."

—*POPULAR SAYING*

Meeting Other Vegetarians

- Check to see if your community has a vegetarian singles group.
- Join local vegetarian groups. In a supportive group, you can feel the relief of being with other people who share some common assumptions about food. Start one, if one doesn't exist in your community.
- Check on-line resources.
- If you are willing to relocate, move to a vegetarian-friendly community such as Berkeley, California; Ithaca, New York; or Madison, Wisconsin, to name a few.

Dating Meat Eaters

At the beginning of a relationship we might minimize what differentiates us—our diet—because love or sex makes it seem possible to do so. We think everything is possible. And we don't want to imagine otherwise. At that moment, as one vegetarian advises: "Think *now* about what life with your meat-eating boyfriend or girlfriend will be like in the future." After all, dating can lead to living together. What is your bottom line for a partner?

Many vegetarians say, "If I had been a vegetarian when I met my partner, the relationship would never have developed." My friend Maria said this even more explicitly:

We are now both sure that if we were to meet each other for the first time with our present diverging beliefs, we would not be interested in having a relationship. Although we obviously have other things that keep us together, eating is a very important part of life, a big part of companionship and community, it is what we do to celebrate and what we do when we mourn and commemorate, so it must play a big role in any decision to live together. We no longer share the comfort of a common meal or the pleasure of a meal prepared together. When I am

147

*low, he cannot help by bringing me a tray of freshly prepared food, nor
can I do this for him.*

What is your bottom line? Some vegans have decided not even to
be friends with meat eaters. Some will be friends, but not sexually intimate, with meat eaters, telling their dates that they won't kiss or physically get close to someone unless they are also vegan, "as their skin,
mouth, bodily fluids, etc. totally gross me out." The bumper sticker says
it all: "Vegetarians taste better." Before the scourge of AIDS and other
sexually transmitted diseases, I observed that being a vegan seems to
sanctify lovemaking because the only body fluids of another animal that
you interact with are those of your lover. Now we can still believe this,
but protecting oneself from infectious diseases is essential. Vegetarianism
should mean that you are committed to taking care of yourself. Extend
this caretaking to other areas of your life. If you are sexually active, be
sure to protect yourself against unplanned pregnancies and sexually
transmitted diseases.

If dating is leading to something more long term, do:

1. Negotiate before you begin living together. Don't assume that
appropriate resolutions to differences will simply evolve. Will there be
meat in the house? How will the refrigerator be arranged? Will there
be separate cookware if there is meat in the house? Is your partner careful about where meat is put, and does your partner clean up carefully?
Will any potential children follow your diet or your partner's?

One woman gave a copy of *The Sexual Politics of Meat* to a man she
had started dating. She told him, "If you want to understand me, you
need to read this book." He did, became a vegan, and moved across the
country to live with her.

2. Know your bottom line. For instance, I knew that raising vegetarian children was very important to me. One way to identify your
bottom line is to recognize what you hold to in other friendships and
relationships. Is this relationship with your partner asking you to sus-

pend something that you would never do in other less intense and committed relationships?

3. Be alert to how the difference in food choices absorbs or displaces other disagreements. Or vice versa, how other disagreements absorb or displace these differences. Are you able to talk honestly about having different approaches to eating?

4. Know what is worth trading. A change in household responsibilities in return for the prospective partner's trying vegetarianism? Perhaps the partner offers a deal: "I'll do this, you do that." "I'll be vegetarian, while you give me x, y, or z." Or you offer the deal to your partner. It has to be something that is equally important to the partner and it has to be an exchange of activities that is parallel. Perhaps "I won't eat meat in the house if I can watch the ballgame uninterrupted on the weekends."

LOVING A MEAT-EATING PARTNER

Vegetarians are often seen as inflexible and controlling. We may see meat eaters in this same light. Intimate relationships, however, must be grounded on love not control, flexibility not inflexibility. As with much of life, we must learn the art of balancing.

I have met many people who stayed blocked vegetarians because they believed their partner needed to eat meat. They have not known how to envision any other arrangement. But there is one: change and tell your partner you changed. Relationships can handle change. Thwarted desires, secrets, self-sacrificial behavior with nothing in return, and fear of change—these can be enormous stressors in relationships. The poet Rainer Maria Rilke talks of a good marriage (and I'll expand it to any long-term committed partnership) as one in which "each appoints the other the guardian of his solitude." There is growth we need to do for ourselves, through solitude, not only for the relationship. We have to allow each other the grace to change, to grow inwardly. Sometimes this inward growth leads to vegetarianism.

What Is Intimacy?

Intimacy requires that we be able to hear and empathize with the partner. Our vegetarianism may mean that we do not want to hear them, and we cannot empathize with them in this one area of their lives. Is your vegetarianism, or your partner's meat eating, influencing your ability to be intimate as a couple?

- Does the relationship allow you to be who you are?
- Does the relationship allow your partner to be who he or she is?
- Can you talk openly about important matters?
- Can you discuss your differences about eating in an even tone?
- Do you know where you stand on emotional issues and can you say so to your partner?
- Are you each able to identify what is acceptable and tolerable in the relationship and what is unacceptable and intolerable?
- Are you able to stay emotionally connected to the other partner even though they think, feel, believe, and eat differently than you do?
- Can you accept your partner without needing to change, convince, cajole, or fix them?

Pressure Points in Intimate Relationships

The more that vegetarianism is now or becomes an expression of the deepest part of you (beliefs about spirituality, the self, ethics), the more you may have to silence that self in relationship to a meat-eating partner. That may be fine for you. You simply need to be aware that this is happening. The relationship with your partner has such depth itself that it also speaks to this deepest part of you. But if you have made any compromises around meat eating by your partner (i.e., fixing it and/or eating it in front of you), you may come to feel that this deepest part is splitting in half. A part is betrayed by your partner's meat eating; a part is supported and enlarged by your partner's love. You have to balance what you feel you are sacrificing in yourself and what you need to sacrifice in the relationship. This is not easy.

But this is precisely where our problems arise.

A woman had become a vegetarian after being married for many years. Now many issues existed in their relationship that had never been there before. After we talked about the frustrations, I asked her what her partner felt about it. What was he going through? She had never thought to ask. That was the next step for her. As Lillian Hellman said, "People change and forget to tell each other." Intimate relationships require openness to change and to hearing about change. But there will be pressure points that occur because of change. Some of them may be:

- You want your partner to change. The problem, of course, is that you cannot change your partner. This isn't easy to accept. If you don't accept that you cannot change your partner, you may be disappointed. Then you will blame the meat-eating partner not only for being a meat eater but for your feeling of disappointment.

- Your partner may see you, at times, as controlling. If your partner says, "I feel oppressed by your vegetarianism," you need to be able to hear what the partner is feeling and why. If your partner is not sufficiently in touch with his or her emotions to be able to articulate this, but is acting in ways that communicate it (edginess, combativeness about choosing dinner or restaurants, inflexibility in some area), the actions communicate this same statement.

- When your partner needs your love because they are sick, you give them a lecture on their diet. They think they have the flu, but you just "know" it is salmonella poisoning. Just as some people blame any illness we might have on our diet, we, similarly, may blame any illness meat eaters have on *their* diet. Though we might be on firmer ground, judgment is still offered as a substitute for loving. This is most unpleasant to someone needing nurturance.

- A time will come when you may announce, "I don't want to make love to you because of your meat eating." Do you say it because it's true, or are you using it as an excuse to cover some other issue? The partner will respond and, besides being hurt, knows full well that you yourself have habits that could come under scrutiny. Maybe it's not meat eating, but to the partner it is as important to them as your vegetarianism is to you.

- Do you fill up the emotional space available for vegetarianism? Vegetarians need to ask: Would my partner be a vegetarian if it weren't for me? We actually keep them from exploring it because we have filled the common space with our version of vegetarianism and they can't find theirs. The meat-eating partner may have no space to discover his feeling or thoughts about vegetarianism separate from his relationship to his partner. The partner may feel she is losing the ability to define herself.

One friend told me:

I lived with my then boyfriend (now husband) when he was a meat eater for several years before he became nearly vegan, and I am certain that I delayed his transition. I simply could not tolerate his meat eating, even though he didn't eat animals in our home or in front of me, and I was constantly interrogating him: "What did you have for lunch? Why did you eat that?" I was insufferable. I have since learned many other, more effective techniques that do not set people up to dig in their heels defensively. Eventually, I decided not to ask him anymore, and casually left literature in key spots around the house (the dining-room table and the bathroom specifically). Whether it was the literature, or my shift in attitude and behavior, six months later, he gave up meat. What I learned from this is that while it can be horribly upsetting and nearly intolerable to endure meat eating among people close to me, my response to those people largely determines whether or not they begin the transition to a more cruelty-free diet. It was as if I had been a really bad lawyer representing my client, the animals, while they needed a much more astute, clever, and detached attorney. Of course, to do this means that I must live in a "role" and not feel or express my own emotions.

- Are you trying to punish your partner for the world's meat eating? Say you see a cattle truck on its way to the slaughterhouse—your feelings might include outrage, sadness, powerlessness. In that cattle truck you see the painful reminder of so many reasons to become a vegetarian. You may also feel bitter, sensing how little has changed. Where does this feeling of powerlessness, of bitterness, this sense that the outer world got to you again, go? Unless you are careful, your partner may become the target, because he represents that world to you. The meat-eater partner then carries the weight of the meat-eating world's sins on his back.

- Can you make deals? (see discussion under "Know what is worth trading," page 149). What trade can you live with or offer? What trade would you feel compromises you? Make a list of activities and behaviors that are in conflict for each of you or things you would prefer your partner did or didn't do. Then negotiate from that list.

A mixed relationship may thrive if both individuals have no control issues and are extremely flexible. But most of us are not so wise in life, and we find that we are at times petty, judgmental, and needy. It is our partners who make us feel secure when we feel insecure, attended to when we feel neglected, loved when we feel unloved. But conflicts with partners are inevitable. It may be because of a disagreement with them that we are feeling insecure, neglected, and unloved. At those times when the relationship is most stressed, meat-eating–vegetarian issues will increase in strength. We need to be aware of this.

Conflicts

Do you each discover new ways to offend each other? The pattern pre-exists your vegetarianism, but your vegetarianism receives the negative energy that hasn't been dealt with. One friend, Marta, told me, "The things I might forgive in a vegetarian partner, I find unforgivable in a meat-eating partner." Meat eating increased interpersonal tensions. She was less tolerant overall because she was so alert to his meat eating. Once she realized that she was judging him in other areas for his meat eating, Marta determined not to confuse her disappointment about her partner's diet with her disappointment about something extraneous to it.

You may discover that something new in the relationship is bothering you. Your partner has started to behave in a certain way that concerns you. You don't feel comfortable confronting your partner about this behavior. Yet you feel edgy, unhappy, disconcerted by it. You will respond by trying to find a place where the other partner is already vulnerable. Finally, you snap at your partner and complain about something safe, something already "on the table," his or her meat eating.

Sexual relationships may become the focus of your meat-eating–vegetarian conflicts. "How can I make love to a person who has just eaten meat? You smell and taste different." If you have that feeling, be aware of it. Don't deny it. It will figure in your relationship if you aren't honest with it.

You may take the other's diet personally: "You are rejecting me in rejecting my food." Suddenly an argument arises. Be careful! Remember, incompatibility does not arise from differences, it arises from whatever prompts them to stand out. What is causing the differences to be more serious at this point than earlier in the week? Are you or your partner tired? Is it the full moon? Are you recovering from a taxing visit of your boss/parents/noisy neighbors?

You balance relationship needs by *knowing your bottom line and clari-*

fying your expectations. But intimate relationships require that you identify and understand your partner's basic needs and also what your partner can and cannot give up. Identify and understand what you can give up without violating your bottom line.

If you are feeling embattled all the time in the relationship, then conflict is exposing incompatibility. A serious stressor is affecting your relationship. It needs your attention. Recall a time when vegetarianism wasn't an issue. What was working then that doesn't work now? The relationship at that point was giving you both something that it isn't giving you now. What was it? Intimacy? Support? Honesty? Casualness about food? Respect? Sexual freedom? At some point you minimized differences that now are painful. Have you changed more than you thought? Can you tolerate a meat-eating partner? Or is vegetarianism carrying the burden of a different—and perhaps to the relationship, a more dangerous—disagreement? The pressure is on you to determine this.

HOW WILL WE RAISE OUR CHILDREN?

You are a vegetarian. Your partner is not. How will you raise your children? Clarify your feelings and make your decisions as much as possible before having children. Different options exist:

The children eat meat.
The children are vegetarian.
The children eat vegetarian at home but eat meat outside the
    house.

I often hear, "I plan on having children with my lover, who is a meat eater. Vegetarianism is very important to me. Should I agree that they can eat meat?"

This is what I tell them: It may feel difficult to know what will be best for you and your children before you have any. That is because love believes all things are possible. Baby poop will teach you otherwise.

Beware of promises that are made in the absence of actual knowledge about a situation. When that meat-eating baby is your responsibility, you may find yourself begrudging the promise. Now you are experiencing the day-to-day demands that feeding a child involves. No matter how much you negotiate how this will actually occur, at some point feeding your children meat or packing their lunches may fall within your responsibility. How will you feel about that?

You may find that this responsibility comes to represent every negative aspect that strains your relationship. Raising children provokes stress anyway—sleep deprivation, discovering old issues from your childhood, the conflict between child raising and work. Adding to that mix an act of parenting that may conflict with your own principles (whether they be motivated by issues of health, the environment, or ethics), puts a great deal of pressure on you. You may discover that petty issues loom larger. A question that might have been innocent—"What are you preparing for supper?"—is suddenly burdened with conflicting expectations. You may begrudge a promise made when you were ignorant of its ramifications, now that you are not able to get out of it.

As your own experience might have shown you, it is easier to *be* someone than to *become* someone else. From your children's perspective, it is easier for them to be vegetarian than to become vegetarian later on. They are not blocked or unblocked, simply free from meat. Not only is it healthier but they can be at peace with their vegetarianism, not having been exposed to a competing diet that infuses taste buds. And they don't beg you to go to McDonald's for a Happy Meal or for the toy prize. This is a constant frustration for some vegetarian parents I know.

It is better to negotiate a vegetarian diet for your children and to do so long before unprotected sex imposes a deadline for the negotiation. It is, after all, a gift to the kids. Besides, the baby poop of meat-eating babies *is* an overwhelming smell. Each diaper may assail you with your dietary differences.

The negotiation involves acknowledging something that is equally as important for your partner as your vegetarianism is to you. My partner and I decided that our children would have his last name and my diet. Not only did this preserve equality, but it provides a one-liner to explain your family's arrangements. In essence, it says, "We have worked this out. You do not need to be worried" to all of those individuals outside of your relationship who will assume they can have opinions on the matter.

The meat-eating world—and your partner—can accommodate your child's vegetarianism. It may not always be easy, but in the long run it is easier than your accommodating a child's meat eating. If your partner has some real concerns in this area, you may not be ready to have unprotected sex until those concerns are more closely examined. A conflict deeper than you realize may exist. Meat eating may represent something to your partner that is more central than you two may have acknowledged. Find this out now, before you have to change a diaper.

Raising Vegetarian Children

If you and your partner agree to raise vegetarian children, and unless you live in a vegetarian commune, raising vegetarian children involves a constant process of mediating your best interests for your child with a meat-eating world, which seems poised to bulldoze them over in an instant if your attention lapses.

You will inevitably get involved in conversations about your vegetarianism with other parents:

Meat eater: "What about your children?"
You: "They're vegetarian, too."
Meat eater: "But do you think it is fair that they didn't have a choice?"
You: "Did your children have a choice?"

Once children are in the picture, the problem becomes trusting relatives to respect their diet. Suddenly your parents are screaming "child abuse" because you are not feeding your children meat. What should you do?

Give them Virginia Messina and Mark Messina's *The Vegetarian Way* and ask them to read the pertinent chapters. Tell them you will discuss the issue with them once they have read it. If they don't read it, that will tell you that no matter what they say, they don't really think the issue is nutritional. If it isn't nutritional, then what they are enacting is an intense resistance. Reread the section on resistance tactics (pages 137–145), and anticipate that your parents will give you an extremely hard time. This may include feeding them foods that you have asked them not to feed them. They are trying to reestablish control.

When your child will be eating out with others or at someone else's house, review with the adults involved what is and is not acceptable as food. Once the child is five or so, they know how to reject meat. By the time they are nine or so, they can negotiate even the esoteric issues of chicken stock in gravy, etc.

Give individuals one chance and one chance only. If they feed your child meat, they have revealed themselves as untrustworthy. If these individuals happen to be members of your family, you have a real problem. They have experienced you as deviating from the family system. This is threatening to them. They have never experienced you as deviating from the family system so completely. They want to bring you back in line and will use your children to do so. Know your bottom line. Betrayal by your parents is not acceptable. Remember that most grandparents want to be with their grandchildren. Let them understand very clearly: "I love you, Mom and Dad. But you must respect my decision on this. If you cannot respect my decision, you are telling me that I can't trust you. What model do you provide my children if you are disrespectful of their parents? Let me show you all the wonderful food they can eat. Then show me that I can trust you. Otherwise, the kids will not stay with you unless I am with them." This may feel very tough, but it often succeeds in communicating your bottom line and from there negotiating something acceptable to you and your parents.

Cooking with Children

Whether you raise your children as vegetarians or meat eaters, be sure to involve them in kitchen activities. Let your children learn how to cook. Your partner and you can supervise their cooking. When my children were in preschool they loved to help with baking. By the time they are in school, if not before, they can help measure ingredients. Children eight and nine can be washing vegetables, mixing, chopping, baking, reading recipes. Children ten to twelve can plan, prepare, and clean up a meal on their own. Teenagers can help plan the menu and shop for groceries as well as cook a meal.

If they are vegetarians, your children need to know how to cook as a survival tactic in this meat-eating world. If they are meat eaters, the more they learn how to cook their favorite foods, the less pressure exists on you.

Give your children the gift of cooking. And, if at all possible, give them the gift of vegetarianism.

11

Grace at Work:
Eating with Meat Eaters

Vegetarians cause chaos. Invited to eat with friends or returning to our family home, we refuse all dishes with animal products and often disconcert our hosts. We are threatening two institutions. Obviously, one is meat eating. The other is the meal itself as it is traditionally experienced. When we decline the traditional foods found at a meal, we throw the meal off by the degree to which everyone believes it requires meat.

Let's face it, it can be uncomfortable eating with meat eaters. Either they are busy thinking about what *we* are doing or we are busy thinking about what *they* are doing. We either cause chaos at their meals or they prompt chaotic emotions within us. Threading our way through conversations and arguments on the one hand, and the ingredients list on the other, we not only feel isolated; we feel frustrated. We feel as though we are in a situation way beyond that of just being controlled. We feel frustrated with our job, our friend, our date, or our family—whoever contributed to our being at this table.

THE RITUAL FUNCTION OF MEALS

Sharing food together confirms that we are a part of the fabric of a community. Weddings, funerals, festival dinners of one sort or another cement relationships, ease transitions, and confirm stability. The way we move forward and the way we remember is through food. When people are ill we take food to them. When we are ill we receive food.

At a meal, the pattern of what is eaten and in what order establishes boundaries. When we eat what is on the table, we are within the boundary. When we don't, we aren't.

In our culture, meat often provides an assurance of continuity and connectedness. It is meat that is the centerpiece, the apex of a meal. The meal builds up to and then down from the main course of meat. Sometimes meals are associated specifically with the animal being consumed: Thanksgiving turkey, Christmas goose in England, Easter ham for Christians, a Fourth of July barbecue. The centerpiece of the meal reassures everyone that they are a group, whether a family, or co-workers, or college friends; it proclaims, "We are in this way the same— we eat the same foods." From this, a circle is drawn and we are all inside it. We feel safe, affirmed, "not different." The meal is a sign of stability: the world may be changing, there may be things out of our control, "but, by God! we can still enjoy a good steak dinner." Or, "Thanksgiving just wouldn't be Thanksgiving without a turkey." The meat confirms social stability. Enter a vegetarian. You are the transgressor. What was stable becomes unstable, what was unquestioned is questioned. The relaxation and exhilaration of the event are strained. What is this individual going to take away from us?

Nobody wants to feel anxious when they eat. Anxiety denies people a feeling of abundance at a meal. When eating is no longer an experience of abundance it loses its deepest rewards.

Meat eaters don't want to feel anxious when they are eating. And meat eaters often feel anxious around vegetarians. Anxiety and eating create tensions. No one benefits from this. People want to enjoy the present moment. People want to feel connected through a meal. The sense that everyone is enjoying the same experience is important. No matter what we do as individuals, our vegetarianism will disrupt this sense of unity. How deep the fissure goes usually depends upon us. If people think, as they talk with us or survey our plate, "What is left for her to give up?" or we discover there is nothing we can eat at communal meals, then the fabric of community is torn.

Yes, we are excluded from meals that were very much a part of our past. But the thing is to start again, to recognize that the food itself is not what is really bringing us together—it is the ritual of eating together. And with this knowledge, we can start working to affirm the abundance of vegetarian foods. The challenge for the vegetarian is to transform chaos into the chaos effect.

FROM CHAOS TO THE CHAOS EFFECT

Thanks to the movie *Jurassic Park,* chaos theory was introduced to the general public. Jeff Goldblum's character explained the "butterfly effect," the idea that a butterfly flapping her wings in Beijing can transform weather systems in New York the next month. Chaos theory provides a way to perceive an order in nature where previously confusion had been seen. Slight deviations are more important than we think. This is why, whenever possible, we should act with this understanding and bring a vegetarian dish to share.

Vegetarian food—one appetizing dish at the Thanksgiving meal, one magnificent salad, one sandwich in the midst of meat, one food that you are happily eating—sends many messages: There is food you can eat. You are not needy, worried, neglected. You have taken care of yourself and seem happy. And your food looks—and tastes—appetizing to others.

Bringing a vegan dish actually accomplishes two things: it ensures that we have something to eat (no small matter!) and it offers nonvegans the chance to try our food. The introduction of one different thing into the scripted meal can have an impact greater than we would think. One dish, for nonvegans, pulls their chaotic, unfocused energies and emotions about veganism into focus. It is about this dish. This *tasty* dish. The vegan is then experienced as connected to the nonvegan—both like tasty food. When we simply cause chaos at the table, we are experienced as different because we are seen only as rejecting foods.

How to Connect at Holiday Meals

- Indulge as many traditions as possible. It creates the feeling of continuity, affirms your connections, speaks to the trained appetite, makes you feel included. You won't miss what is missing as much if you are enjoying everything possible.

- Ask yourself: Given the circumstance of the day, what would make my meal special?

- Make up a title to a recipe that can be specific to the event, like "Aunt Edna's beans." It inaugurates a tradition. Our mind is associative. It likes to put two and two together. Event-related titles for recipes speak to this associative desire. Then we simultaneously feed the person, feed the memory, and feed the mind. We prepare people for the following year, when we bring the same dish.

- Research your cultural heritage and find out what vegetarian foods have always been a part of it. That is exciting and surprising, since so many ethnic traditions could not count on a plentiful supply of meat. Cookbooks are a great help. You may not be eating the meat on the table, but you can remind your family what traditions you still accept and follow.

- If you are invited by a family member who already knows you are a vegetarian, simply say, "I'll bring along my *famous* hoisin tofu or my *famous* nutty salad." With a host who is new to your diet, you can say, "I'm a vegetarian, but don't worry about fixing something special. I would like to bring my *famous* sweet potato soup, tabouli, noodle salad, [etc.]." "Famous" helps establish its credibility as a dish.

Chaos theory explains the irregularities of life—the burst of static on a telephone line, the coastline, lightning bolts. Being trained to see the world as meat eaters, they cannot explain the attractions of our diet. But create a little irregularity in the meal, bring that dish, and they now have a way to grasp it.

Linear dynamics (A causes B, which results in C) cannot explain chaos theory. Neither can it explain the effect of our own dish on those who eat it. That one dish has a greater effect than we can comprehend. It provides an opening to someone else to be receptive. People see wonderful food; they try it. In the process, something unfamiliar becomes familiar.

IT TAKES TWO OF YOU, EVEN IF YOU'RE THE ONLY ONE

Question: How many vegans does it take to change a lightbulb?
Answer: Two—one to change it and one to check for animal ingredients.

It may seem like it takes two of you to eat with meat eaters. One of you must anticipate so that the other can enjoy. You anticipate so that there can be full abundance in your eating experience. Otherwise, you experience scarcity and teach others that their fears about your diet (that there is nothing you can eat) are true. Recall the young woman whose Thanksgiving dinner at her grandmother's consisted only of a toasted bagel. I urged her to see that such a situation was not healthy for her or her family.

But one dish could transform it. She could be having something fancy or something simple. It doesn't matter. The goal is to be able to share and bring others into your world. Until we bring that dish, our world seems to be a world of *not* eating. With that dish, we demonstrate otherwise. We share our contentment.

Yes, there need to be two of you: the planner part of you, who thinks ahead, knowing that the meat-eating world may leave us only a toasted bagel. The planner anticipates in the face of scarcity, so that the eater part of you can know abundance. By the time you sit down to eat, the planner should have done his/her job so that the eater can eat happily, joyfully, knowing only abundance.

Your need to have food you can eat intersects with nonvegetarians' need not to see you as a stranger and to experience your foods. Then they can think to themselves: Maybe there is abundance in this choice, too. There's another reason not to show scarcity. If you aren't eating much, people automatically assume you have an eating disorder—and denial doesn't work. You must prove your ability to eat food and keep it down, if you want to keep the respect of your peers.

It is the planner's responsibility to make sure the answer is yes to the question "Will there be something for me to eat?" There are many ways the planner part of you can assure this. You need to identify which way will meet your needs.

Ways to Plan Ahead: Engaging the Planner Part of You

- Always have a backup plan when eating with meat eaters.
- Eat ahead of time.
- Talk with the host.
- Bring food.

One major problem exists. Are you the type of person who takes your needs seriously enough that you will develop the skills of planning ahead? When you are going to be eating with others, do you say, "Don't worry about me" because you are frightened of being rejected? Some people's tolerance for what they see as calling attention to themselves is so low that they cannot stand the social drama that arises from saying, "I am a vegetarian." They experience that statement as saying, "I have specific needs in this situation, can you assist me?" This feels unbearable. For instance, a friend of mine was chosen to receive an important award from an impressive group at a formal dinner. Although he was the awardee, he made no advance plans with the sponsors to indicate that he would not be eating the main course at the banquet. His uneasiness was unfortunate. Of course the sponsors would want their awardee to be fed. Of course the banquet chef could accommodate vegetarianism. But his tolerance for having a special need, for needing others to respond to it, was so low he could not make the request. He was what communication specialist Virginia Satir calls a "placator"—someone who won't call attention to himself, no matter what. *Not being willing to negotiate and not making any other arrangements means that you are self-denying.* It is important to feel comfortable giving others the opportunity to provide for your vegetarianism. After all, even if it were not in your self-interest, you need to do it for them, to help avoid the awkwardness that occurs when they see you not eating. Moreover, some meat eaters honestly want to honor your diet but don't know how. You could help them to know what to do. You need to give them the opportunity to honor you, knowing also that they might not.

THE SPIRIT OF ABUNDANCE

If the planner did everything possible, yet you sit down to eat with meat eaters, facing, once again, an iceberg-lettuce salad, focus not on the amount of vegetarian food, or the kind of vegetarian food, but the quality of eating vegetarian food. Find abundance even in this.

You never eat the same meal twice. This means that even if you are eating the one hundredth iceberg-lettuce salad of the year in a restaurant, it is an entirely new iceberg-lettuce salad to you that day. Let the moment be that of living in the present and rejoicing in your vegetarianism. At the moment when you are eating the salad, nothing in that restaurant would be better than it, because if it were, you would probably be eating it. So that lettuce salad deserves all your attention for that meal. This gives you a feeling of connection, and feeling connected you can feel abundance. Let us be conscious, even in moments of stress, alienation, or yet again that iceberg-lettuce salad, that we are connected to something unfolding in our lives and in our culture. And remember, the salad itself may carry its own long-term health benefits.

Be Conscious of Your Expectations

You need to be aware of them so that you can be prepared. Do not let your expectations take the place of preparation. Perhaps you are living with an expectation about an upcoming event involving food ("Oh, that will be a great dinner because . . ."). If, for that expectation to be fulfilled, you are relying on the actions of another person, *and* that person does not share your dietary commitments, *you* need to take action and make preparations yourself. Otherwise, you will be living with dashed expectations.

If someone is preparing food for you, be precise about what foods you do not eat—chicken stock, lard, etc. Clarify this with them, while also saying, "I do not expect you to have to prepare this food. Let me bring a dish to share."

Lower Your Expectations

Expectations can keep us from being prepared. After I became a vegan, I stopped expecting that I could eat at most public functions that I was invited to that were not sponsored by vegetarian or animal liberation groups. It was so liberating to lower my expectations! Once I knew I could not expect to be fed, I could enter anyplace without needing to scan for available vegetarian food. The part of me that needs to eat with a feeling of abundance had already done so or was going to after the meal. This was a great gift—the gift of detachment from public meals.

But even if you lower your expectations, you will still be surprised. You cannot anticipate everything.

Let Your Frustrations Teach You

Whenever you find yourself saying, "I'll never put myself through that again!" identify what dynamics need to be changed so that you indeed do not go through it again.

Where was the meal?
What necessity required you to be at the meal?

- Friendship
- Family obligations
- Work requirements
- Social obligations

What specifically occurred that caused the frustration?

- Vegetarian food was promised, but it wasn't there.
- They thought vegetarians ate chicken/fish/lard/chicken stock/anchovies.
- You talked about your vegetarianism.
- Someone ordered on your behalf and you couldn't eat what they ordered.
- Nobody wanted to dine where you wanted to eat.
- You were hungry.
- They would not stop offering you meat.
- You were eating at a restaurant.
- They were eating meat.

Once you identify what has frustrated you, see if there is a pattern to your frustrations. Is it always when you go out to eat? Is it work related or family related? Ask yourself, "How can I avoid this next time?" This requires understanding what sort of power you have in your relationships. You cannot control the behavior of others, but you can keep them from making you a target and you can keep yourself from believing that certain obligatory meals can meet a gustatory need. You need to develop your own ground rules for eating with meat eaters. At a minimum they will probably address the following issues:

Ground Rules for Eating with Meat Eaters

- Don't talk about vegetarianism if meat is present or you are outnumbered.
- If offered meat, say "No thank you."
- When eating outside of your own house, assume nothing.
- Be prepared not to be fed.

- Therefore, BYOF (bring your own food): Create and share vegetarian food as much as possible.
- Be aware of your feelings about someone else's meat eating.

Saying "No Thank You"

If offered meat, you can say, "No thank you." Deny people the opportunity to use your behavior to start an argument. One vegetarian reported, "When in the company of others who have different menu habits from mine, I simply don't eat what I don't want to eat . . . much like a six-year-old. It is always possible to say, 'I'm not hungry, I can grab something to eat later.'"

"Would you like some meat?"

"No thank you."

"Why not?"

"I prefer not to."

"Are you sure?"

"Yes, thank you."

"This concerns me."

"It doesn't need to."

"Are you sure you are okay?"

"Yes. Thank you."

"But I fixed it just for you."

"Thank you, but no thanks."

"Are you sure?"

"Yes, thank you."

"But I worked all day!"

"No thank you."

"Don't you love me?"

"Let's not confuse the issue."

"Once won't hurt, will it?"

"No thanks."

You wish to discourage people from questioning your practices and beliefs. Your desire is to redirect the conversation, to escape being the focus, to be courteous without accepting someone else's agenda. The cook's efforts do not mandate that the food be consumed.

DINING OUT

Restaurants Beef Up Vegetarian Menus
—HEADLINE IN THE *WALL STREET JOURNAL*

You can say that again! They *beef* them up, *chicken* them up, *pig* them up. Well, beef stock, chicken stock, lard them up. We all know that problem.

We all have our own stories of our worst experiences at a restaurant. Having to spit out meat? That's happened. Restaurant staff who don't understand the word *vegetarian?* That too. Recall, in Chapter 1, a salad bar where everything was contaminated with some form of meat or dairy and a steak house where the vegetable was "chicken and biscuits." Those ubiquitous Chinese buffets with . . . well, you know.

When we go out to eat, we want a sense of abundance: "There is something for me to eat that I will enjoy." We want a sense of welcome: "The people I am with enjoy my company, and I enjoy theirs. And the wait staff make me welcome." But who always gets what they want?

Living Among Meat Eaters' Rules for Dining Out

- Don't assume anything about your wait staff (i.e., that they know what *vegetarian* means, that they understand you don't eat foods with chicken stock in it, that they know Parmesan means cheese, that they understand that gelatin, lard, and anchovies are animal products).
- Do as much negotiating as you can with the restaurant on behalf of your needs before arriving there.
- Know your threshold for others' meat eating.
- Eat before you go.

Yes, going out to eat, unless to an explicitly vegetarian restaurant, may seem to have gotten more complicated. But break apart the various aspects of it: who, what, when, and where, and you are on the road to having some control in a situation where loss of control often afflicts us.

1. Do you want to go out to eat? Identify this first. Just because you are invited does not mean you have to go. If you are invited somewhere, instead of feeling that you have to answer immediately, simply say, "I have to check my calendar and get back to you." You don't have to say anything more. That gives you some time to decide if this is what you want to do. If you are invited to go to a restaurant, call that restaurant and find out if they have any dishes that meet your dietary needs. Give yourself some time to think about the value of the event and the demands it will make on you.

2. Do you have a role in selecting the restaurant? If you do, suggest restaurants that you know serve food of a primarily vegetarian style without its being obvious that this is what they do—a Thai restaurant, perhaps, or a Middle Eastern one. As one vegan wrote, "That way I can put up with them and they usually don't even notice that their chickpea curry or falafel is decidedly lacking in meat." You can assume that for the most part you will be able to get a good meal at a Chinese restaurant. Almost every one has a version of Buddha's Delight, which is vegan. Your fallback can be a pizzeria; cheeseless pizzas with vegetables, and a little olive oil drizzled on top, can in themselves be very tasty.

Assess your degree of power in negotiating the choice of restaurant. Don't be naive. If you are relatively powerless, low on the work or family totem pole, you need to recognize this. The sooner the better. Be aware, as well, whether your companions are deliberately not choosing the restaurant that you want. This sort of power dynamic may be at work when they want to thwart your veganism rather than support you. So don't leap into the discussion with your first choice. Simply by being your first choice, it may be the one least likely to be adopted.

What do you do when, for employment, family, or another reason, the group selecting the place to dine is either consciously or unconsciously ignoring your choice in diet?

If you have little individual power to sway a group choice, enlist a meat-eating ally, someone in the loop when decisions are being made, who will help steer the "gang" from some of the least inviting places. Ask this person to help represent your concerns, perhaps suggesting a restaurant where everyone can get meals. When the suggestion comes from someone like them, it isn't seen as a special pleading by the interested party. Therefore it isn't tainted by anyone's feelings about your vegetarianism or you.

If this is a spontaneous event, and your friends or family are supportive, you can go into a restaurant and ask to see their menu, perhaps talking with the maître d' before deciding to eat there. My family waits while I "scout" out a place to ensure its food will be acceptable to all.

3. Do some advance work. If someone else has chosen the restaurant or you have agreed to go to a nonvegetarian restaurant, offer to make the reservations. If you aren't making the reservations, try to learn where you are going beforehand. Then do your advance work.

If you can, check out the Internet. Does your local paper post their restaurant reviews? Does the restaurant itself have a site? If you have a fax machine, have a menu faxed to you. Whether you have these resources or not, call the restaurant at a time when they can answer your questions without being rushed.

Don't just ask, "Do you serve vegetarian food?" and think you are covered, and don't talk just to the maître d'. Ask to speak to the chef or kitchen manager if it is between meals. Cookbook author Ken Haedrich, winner of the Julia Child Cookbook Award, explains: "He or she should be willing and able to talk to you intelligently about the sort of food you would like. And you should get the distinct impression that the chef knows something about meatless cuisine and looks at feeding you as a creative challenge, not as a pain in the patootie. If the chef mumbles something about a baked potato and the salad bar, this is not a good sign." Be very specific about your dietary choice. Say, "I am a vegetarian," and define what you mean, with explicit comments such as "I do not eat land or sea animals." Say whether or not you eat dairy products or eggs. Say, "I want a vegetarian meal that does not have any meat, chicken, fishes, cheese, milk, or eggs in it. This includes no chicken or meat stock, no lard, no anchovies."

You might begin by asking, "What vegetarian entrees do you offer?" This lets them know that at least one person assumes that they should be offering vegetarian entrees. Then ask and be specific in your questions:

Do you put chicken stock in soups or sauces (such as tomato sauces or other sauces that go over pasta)?

Are there eggs in your pasta?

What do you cook your French fries in? Not, Do you cook your French fries in vegetable oil or animal fat? As one vegetarian observed to me, "Some restaurants will tell you whatever they think you want to hear. If you asked them, 'Do you cook them in vampire's blood?' They'd say 'yes.'"

Do you cook your tomato sauce with meat and then strain it out? Don't ask, "Is there meat in the sauce?" They may say no, because there *isn't*. But there *was*. Order the marinara sauce instead.

Does the chef use a meat-based stock for flavoring or thinning?

If there are no vegetarian entrees, you can try to determine if a meat meal can be prepared without the meat. A portobello-mushroom-and-meat sandwich could have the meat left out; a Reuben sandwich made with sauerkraut and avocado instead of meat can be pretty tasty. Pasta with steamed, roasted, or grilled vegetables in an olive oil–garlic sauce is good. Combine a set of side dishes and/or appetizers into your own specialized vegetable plate. And yes, if necessary, a baked potato with ingredients from the salad bar topping it.

See if you can create from their usual ingredients a meal that you can look forward to and that they can make. The more formal and expensive a restaurant, the more likely that they will be equipped to meet your requests. Reach an agreement with them about what can be ordered, and be sure to write down the names of the people with whom you talked. Then at dinner you can say, "I spoke with Theresa the chef this afternoon, and she indicated that she could prepare roasted vegetables with fennel seeds and balsamic vinegar and baked tofu."

4. If circumstances have not allowed you to pick the restaurant or make advance plans, try to keep as much of the negotiation out of sight as possible. Excuse yourself from the table, go to the kitchen or the maître d', and find out about vegan options. This spares embarrassment for people who aren't used to asking the server questions about what is in their meal. If you ask questions in front of a mixed group, your questions about food choices will make the others feel uneasy, while providing them with another example of why they couldn't be vegetarians. (They think, "Who would want to submit themselves to that just to go out to eat and relax? Where's the relaxation in that?") Indeed, this may be one of the reasons the meat eater is blocked. Meat eaters are often discomforted by what they consider the tedious ritual that vegetarians must run through when ordering at a restaurant. They may not like doing anything that calls attention to themselves, and from their perspective, this "inquisition" of the wait staff is embarrassing. The result is that they think, "I could never become a vegan because I could never go through that." Of course, they may be the very same people who, when your meal arrives, exclaim, "Oh I wish I had ordered that."

5. Do what you have to do to avoid having to send a dish back. There is something excruciating about sitting without food in front of you when everyone else is eating. Either they feel self-conscious about eating and wait for you while their food gets cold, or you encourage them to eat and they feel awkward about it. You are aware of them eating or not eating. You become more aware of what they are eating, too. Your apparent confrontation with the wait staff in sending the food back may make them uncomfortable. No matter what you say, you are calling attention to yourself.

But if you have to, send it back. If there is something suspicious about the food when it arrives, ask questions. This, of course, is the most difficult time for you to discover that communication was not what you thought it was. But, hey, better late than never.

6. And, if you think the place you are going to cannot in *any* way accommodate you and yet you *must* go: eat before you go.

7. Let restaurants know what you think. Appendix C at the back of this book is a "Vegetarian Patrons of Restaurants Card." Make multiple copies. Then fold it so that it fits into your wallet. After eating at a restaurant, fill it in and leave it for the management and the chef. If you go to restaurants because they serve vegetarian food, let them know. And if you get a great meal, let the chef know. As Ken Haedrich explains, "Chefs are not known for their small egos; the more you can express your gratitude for a job well done, the better the kitchen is going to take care of you. Tell them you appreciate their efforts. If you do, tell them you feel strongly about supporting places that cater to vegetarians; then tell your friends. Don't be afraid to drop specific hints about the sort of vegetarian foods you like and *would love to try* if the chef ever made anything like that. Most good chefs like a challenge and they'll do everything they can to keep you happy."

8. Besides letting the establishment and the chef know you enjoyed your meal, think about coming back and spreading the word to your friends. Above all, be sure to tip fairly and appreciatively. You represent a class of people, "vegetarians," and so your actions will reflect on everyone else who also call themselves vegetarians.

GETTING YOUR KIND OF FOOD AT THEIR KIND OF PLACE

- Traveling? Stock a vegetarian survival bag. Carry packets of instant ramen noodles; granola stocked with dried fruits; a plastic jar of peanut butter; small packages of soy, almond, or rice milk; nutritional yeast; instant hummus; canned vegetarian sandwich spreads; instant-soup cups and hot-cereal cups.

- Airlines: When you order your meal on an airline, get the person's name. Always, always, always confirm twenty-four hours ahead of time. But still, don't assume you'll actually get the vegetarian meal you asked for. Any number of things can get between you and your meal—and often do. Give feedback to the flight attendants; they fill out a "comments" card and can often be enlisted to convey your perspective on your behalf. If, after ordering one, there is no special meal available, you can request that they give you coupons that can be used at the airport to get food you can eat.

- School cafeterias. Assume nothing. From preschool to high school, the choices may be very limited. Bringing lunches will be the best option. If you wish to make some changes, contact EarthSave and find out about their school-lunch campaign. Colleges and universities are slowly making vegetarian food available. Most now have vegetarian or animal advocacy groups that work to expand vegan offerings. The main problem is limited choices. Get involved at the administration level before a new contract is signed with the company that manages the food service for your college or university. Ask that bids include vegan entrees. The change might not come in time for you to benefit from this, but future vegan students will be extremely thankful.

- Picnics, barbecues, fish fries. These are often the most difficult because of the smells. Bring your own food. Stay as far away from the cooking action as possible.

- Banquets and other catered events. It is surprising, but these events are often the most flexible. You need to decide on a case-per-case basis whether you need to request your special meal ahead of time. If you do, you need to work through the person who has invited you. If you arrive at the event without having found out about the menu, ask the server to replace the meat with extra vegetables.

- Traveling abroad: Study cookbooks from countries you are going to visit, and list the names of vegetable dishes that sound attractive. They may not be listed on the menus of the restaurants when you visit that country, but the chef may be happy to comply with your vegetarian needs. Check out Bryan Geon's *Speaking Vegetarian: The Globetrotter's Guide to Ordering Meatless in 197 Countries,* or www.vegdining.com, an online guide to vegetarian restaurants around the world. Also, copy the International Vegetarian Card from The Physicians Committee for Responsible Medicine that you can find in Appendix D.

EATING WITH MEAT EATERS WHO ARE EATING MEAT

We have restored the hole in the conscience, meat eaters haven't. How do we respond to their eating dead animals?

Ask yourself, "What do I feel when I watch people eat meat?"

1. It doesn't bother me. I think that that is their choice.
2. I still miss meat.
3. It upsets me greatly: I feel sad and withdraw or I feel angry and want to confront them.

If your answer was #1, you don't have a problem. You can skip this section. You are like Annette:

"If I make the decision to dine with meat eaters, then I accept the consequences. The alternative is not to dine with them—however, I have some very good friends who eat meat. I am not willing not to dine with them—so I practice acceptance, order my vegan meal and am living proof that the vegetarian/vegan lifestyle is a 'happy' choice."

If your answer was #2, you may still be in transition. Many vegetarians advise not eating with meat eaters during this time. Others recommend making sure that you have your comfort foods available. Eat before you go. Remind yourself why you are a vegetarian during the meal.

If you answer #3, you have a problem similar to the vegetarians quoted below.

"The most problematic issue of dining with meat eaters is seeing raw meat being eaten or bones of animals; both just make me want to be physically sick."

"It makes me upset to see my friends eating dead animals, but at the same time they are my friends, so I cannot get angry with them. I feel very conflicted. I don't know if I am going to take it too far one day and cause my friends to not want to be around me if I argue with them every time they eat."

For many, it is simply untenable, unimaginable, to sit by as someone else eats meat. Too much shutting down of your system has to happen for this interaction. It is exhausting. Should we have to partition the fact of what they are doing from our mind? Can we? Why should we let people off the hook? The meat itself assails you—smells, the fact of meat production, everyone's insensitivity, the sight of it. You feel yourself being sacrificed to a communal experience that you don't agree with. Finding yourself feeling disturbed, upset, angry, alienated, how do you respond?

Your choice is avoidance, confrontation, detachment, or meditation.

Avoidance

Whenever possible, avoid eating with meat eaters at nonvegetarian restaurants or in other nonvegetarian circumstances. To avoid feelings associated with watching people eating meat at holiday dinners or cookouts, wait until the meal is over and then arrive. Call first to confirm that the meal is done.

Avoiding watching meat eaters eating meat is often the most difficult goal to achieve. We do not always have this degree of control in our lives. The next-best alternative is that if you are at a meal at someone's house, you might try to sit as far away from the "main course" as possible.

Others handle this problem by establishing a bottom line. They will dine with meat eaters except when at a function or a restaurant where baby calves are being served. They believe that at this point, a consensus should exist that at the minimum, flesh called "veal" is unacceptable.

Confrontation

Nothing we do will revive the dead animal on the table before us. Discussing the animal's death may actually sacrifice the animal again. Blocked vegetarians may dig their heels in even deeper, to become more rigid. The result is that more animals may be lost.

If you cannot live with yourself without speaking up on behalf of the animals, confront gently. Use a one-liner. It's out there and then it's gone. One person explains, "I apologize to what's on their dinner plate. It usually makes them laugh." It gives this individual a coping device, it is based on a sense of justice, and it is integrated, slightly, into the relationship. But remember this: If you get upset about the meat at the table, this reaction teaches meat eaters that even if they become a vegetarian they will be aware of meat. They may think, Why bother?

Detachment

You are upset. First, become aware of what you are feeling. Let the feelings exist, don't deny their legitimacy, but don't let them influence your behavior. Observe them instead. Ask yourself, "What am I feeling?" "Am I feeling angry?" "Am I feeling upset?" Identify the feelings by naming them: "I am angry. I am upset. I am hurt." Ask yourself, "Why am I feeling this feeling?" Your answer might be "Because my friends and family are ignoring what they are doing." Feelings are a state of mind. To begin to name what you are feeling begins to dispel the power of its hold on you. That is the first step, awareness. Second, identify what responses are available to you. You know what is going on now, you are responding to the actions of others over whom you have no power. But what can you do? Learn how to take the jumble of chaotic feelings and focus upon them so that you can acknowledge them and let them be released. You can excuse yourself from the table, or you can do a detachment exercise. To begin, deepen your breathing.

> I breathe in, and am aware of anger [or impatience, despair, violation, frustration—whatever unpleasant emotion that you are feeling] within.
> I breathe out, knowing that this anger, [impatience, despair] is not me.
> I breathe in, aware that anger [or impatience, despair, etc.] is unpleasant.
> I breathe out, I know this feeling will pass.
> I breathe in, feeling my breath calm me.
> I breathe out, aware that this anger need not become me.
> I breathe in, knowing that I am breathing in.
> I breathe out, knowing that I am breathing out.
> I breathe in, breathing to all of me, every finger, every toe, every pore.
> I breathe out, breathing out from every finger, every toe, every pore.
> I breathe in, loving fingers and toes and lungs.
> I breathe out, loving people and cooks and animals.

Continue breathing in and breathing out, slowly, with deep, steady breaths, focusing on moving your feeling from being possessed by anger to feeling calm and centered.

Meditation

If watching people eat meat upsets you, and you are unable to avoid eating with them, practice this meditation before you go. The planner part of you has to take time to prepare for this encounter, so that when you are eating with them, you can call upon this resource.

The purpose of this meditation is to affirm connections, with your health, with the animals, with the environment, with other vegetarians. Its purpose is not to desensitize. It involves concentrating energy before you eat, so that the feelings you have when you are eating and see people eating meat have been addressed prior to that experience, not at the time of the experience. It's another way of being prepared.

Before you go to dinner, take ten minutes. First, identify what bothers you most in eating with meat eaters. Find a way to name it: are there predators in conversation? Is it the meat eating itself? Is it the smells? Is it a feeling of being ignored or neglected? Is it the thought of the animal lying dead before you? Is it your powerlessness? Sit comfortably, with your back straight. Breathe deeply. Establish calmness, by breathing in a rhythmic way.

Say:
Breathing in, I am thankful for my vegetarianism.
Breathing out, I feel centered by my vegetarianism.
Breathing in, I am at peace.
Breathing out, I share my peace with all beings.
Continue this rhythmic breathing for several minutes.

Identify a trigger, a way of reestablishing this sense of calm and wholeness and connectedness. For instance, you might want to bring the index finger and thumb of one hand together in a circle. A gesture such as this is inconspicuous at a dinner table. You can simply rest your hand on your thigh under the table. As you breathe deeply, affirm that at any time you make that gesture, you have the ability to detach from the environment that you are in the midst of and reconnect to this feeling of peacefulness. When you are at the meal with meat eaters, resume the hand position that you used when meditating before the meal.

Recall that feeling you had of gentleness to help focus your emotions on larger connections.

Another preparatory action you can take, in alliance with this one or on its own, is to select an aromatherapy scent that you find calming. Apply a very small amount under your nostrils just before you leave for the meal. When you inhale, those smells will help counter the smells that assail you.

THE GRACE OF THE CHAOS EFFECT

When you bring one vegetarian food item, or more, to a potluck or a family celebration, or order a vegetarian meal at a restaurant, you are able to ignore what meat eaters are eating because you have created something nourishing and life-affirming. You are the butterfly flapping her wings. That vegetarian dish, in and of itself, may start the reorienting process.

There is always a benefit we can't see.

A friend described his Thanksgiving experience. One year when everyone arrived for Thanksgiving dinner at his mother's, there was a note on the blackboard: "This year's meal is vegetarian because so many of the family are now vegetarian." All those vegetarian butterflies in China had flapped their wings, and now, several years later, the meal was transformed. One uncle sat through the entire meal, pouting, refusing to eat anything because there was no turkey. Not even a toasted bagel would he eat! What a loss! That poor uncle! Even though vegetarian food included him, he could not tolerate the idea of eating it. Now he experienced scarcity in the midst of vegetarian abundance.

Small changes over time have a cumulative effect.

One vegetarian played on a baseball team. After ballgames the team always went for pizza. Without saying anything, he ordered a cheeseless veggie pizza. His teammates noticed how good it looked, and asked a few questions, but he deflected a discussion and simply enjoyed his pizza; as they enjoyed theirs. Some asked to taste his pizza and were pleasantly surprised. One of them had high cholesterol and began ordering a cheeseless pizza as well. Another team player had been ordered to cut down on fat because of his arteries. He, too, got a cheeseless pizza. Within a few years, without much focused discussion on veganism per se, the whole baseball team had practically adopted the vegan's diet.

Create the chaos effect, one dish at a time. This allows grace to work.

12

On the Job: Working with, for, and (Sometimes) Against Meat Eaters

From Mike, a law student:

> *At my previous job, we had a central small "kitchen" or lunch area. On several occasions a number of us would be there preparing our lunches and as others bit happily into their hot dogs or luncheon meats that contained an interminable list of ingredients, many of which were unrecognizable or even unpronounceable, they would look at the veggie dog or TVP (etc.) that I was preparing and say, "EEEEEEEWWWWW! What is that? How can you eat that?"*

A work environment can be supportive or backstabbing, cooperative or competitive, nurturing or toxic. Add vegetarianism to the mix and the lunchroom—a place of retreat from the workspace—becomes a combat zone. We threaten meat eaters, yes, but unfortunately for us, we also threaten company camaraderie. Bonding of employees often happens around meals . . . and then we come along. Sometimes everyone bonds *against* us.

It is worth remembering that the word *capital* comes from the root word for *cattle*. In declining the company's foods we throw off our relationship with our co-workers by the degree to which they or the event or the company itself is committed to meat eating. This can mean a difficult work environment for us. Will people trust us? Listen to us? Will it influence the ability of others to evaluate us? Can we succeed at a job if we are not seen as company players?

One woman wrote me about her work environment:

I have been a vegetarian for two years now. I feel that it has been one of the most rewarding decisions that I have made. I have a co-worker who has made the decision to become a vegetarian. There have been so many jokes about us. Because her last name is Brown, they call her "Brown and Serve." I admit that it is sort of funny, but damaging. How do you suggest we defend our choices?

At this point, you are probably equipped to recognize that those co-workers are defensive and so they are releasing their feelings in this way. My advice to her is probably predictable at this point:

Just ignore them. Smile at them. Go on eating your sprouts, your sandwiches, your soups. Ignore them and attribute it to bad manners. The less they can make "you" and your vegetarianism the issue, the more likely it is that they will actually experience what it means to be a vegetarian. You don't have to answer their questions, and you don't have to get sucked into their agenda. Simply smile and change the subject.

Many vegetarian workers discover to their dismay that meat eating is deeply embedded in many assumptions about work. Some discover that their co-workers are saboteurs. One co-worker intentionally left his leather jacket on a vegan's belongings so that she had to touch the leather jacket to get her things. It is okay to make our preferences clear. When she discovered a pattern to his actions, she could have said, "I find it very unpleasant to remove your leather jacket from my belongings." If they persist you could say, even-toned and unemotionally, "I have said that I don't like handling leather. That was rather insensitive." If they persist, say, with the same even tone, "I have said that I don't like handling leather. That was rather mean." It may persist, but then you (if you insist on drawing a line here) should persist with the same observation: that it was mean.

Alternatively, you may ask them to promise not to do this in the future. If they persist, you may remind them, in an even tone, of the promise. Don't be hostile. But if the vegetarian has too many requirements (e.g., no one is allowed to eat flesh in their presence) they will find themselves alienated and unhappy, and these feelings make poor vehicles for spreading vegetarianism.

Many of the problems you encounter at work can be addressed by drawing on the analysis and responses discussed in the previous chapters. Teasing through food is usually a variation of the hostile saboteur. The leather jacket guy is a saboteur. Questions about what you eat or don't eat can be responded to according to the guidelines for talking with meat eaters. Draw on the survival skills of the previous chapters and apply them to this situation. But in addition there are some unique situations in a work relationship that require our attention.

TEAM BUILDING: ITS IRRATIONAL ASPECTS

Are you a team player? Companies need team players. To determine that their employees are team players, they often use a "loyalty" test. This test, which is not explicitly called a test, and is not like any tests that you have taken in school, is often a humiliating experience. You have to pass this one test to be seen as a team player, and then, when it's over, you are never subjected to a similar sort of humiliation again. Team building is about your powerlessness.

No matter how you behave in relationship to your work duties, your vegetarianism may be saying, "I'm not a team player."

The most painful experience I have heard is from a vegan who discovered that the meal she was expected to attend was at a "pick your own lobster house." I'll let her tell the story:

I sat through dinner eating only a portobello mushroom sliver and a side salad (all that was available) while everyone passed oysters, shrimp, caviar . . . and then excused themselves while they went to pick out their lobster (and when they were brought to the table, everyone proceeded to crack jokes like, "Wait a minute, you got Susie, she was the one I picked!"). Everyone ordered steak tartare, veal, etc., and they were all passing the flesh back and forth sharing. All through dinner, they made comments like, "This steak is so tender," or "This is the best cut of meat I have ever had." Everyone at that table knew how I felt about eating animals, yet they continued to make these comments. I sat there, silent, something I never do, which made me feel even worse. It was a horrible night and made me feel very defeated. I almost walked out of the place—what would you have done?

Many signs exist that this was a loyalty test—not just for her but for everyone. The first sign is that it is in an unusual setting: she and her co-workers had all been flown to Tampa. The second sign that this is a loyalty test is that none of them had input into the place they were to eat: the client had chosen a very famous meat-and-seafood place. As the vegetarian woman explained to me, "My boss told me where we were going to be eating, and I thought it was a joke. He is very sympathetic to my lifestyle and he, along with my co-workers, have told me how much they respect and admire the way I live my life—so that was why I was so surprised about where we were to eat. I thought it was very insensitive—my boss could have suggested we go somewhere with a little more variety, but did not." Clearly, in this situation, not even the boss felt that he could challenge the client's choice, despite his sympathies for her position. That was the boss's loyalty test to his client.

During the dinner these usually respectful and admiring co-workers do not ask her how she is enjoying the meal; in fact, their behavior furthers the violation of the environment. Here is the third sign that it is a loyalty test—behavior that is out of character. The fourth sign reveals why: the comments about the food are directed to the most important person present—the client—and to the person who represents the client's interests, the boss. The comments are flowing in a vertical system that moves upward. That is why the steak was "the best they had ever eaten." (In this situation it had to be!) And this is why there were jokes about the poor lobsters.

With a loyalty test in a meat-eating environment, the vegan is the least powerful person there. And even she behaved out of character. She told me she wanted "to open my (usually big) mouth and ask that a little consideration be shown to me." Yet she did not, another sign that the meal was fitting the pattern of a loyalty test. She also reported, "I refuse to be silent." But in this case she did choose silence. She understood that something was different about this meal. What was the difference? She might not have had a conscious label for it (i.e., "This is a loyalty test"), but she understood that something was important enough to keep her there and keep her quiet. She bemoaned the lack of interaction and compassion for her: "I just wished someone would have asked me about my food choices that night, because I would have opened my mouth then." But of course no one could ask her—the flow was toward the powerful, not the powerless. She admits that she was tempted to leave, but she didn't. What held her there? Her loyalty to her boss.

Now some vegetarians believe that she could have said something like:

Listen, folks, if I may get a word in edgewise. I have no intention of spoiling your fun or telling you what to eat. But I wonder if you could show just a little respect for me. It just so happens that I consider eating animals offensive. It offends my personal set of values. I do understand that you don't share my values, and that's fine. But I'm sure, if I were Jewish, you would refrain from telling jokes about Jews, out of respect for me. And so, if you don't mind, perhaps we could just cut down a little on joking about all these dead animals and talk about something else. I'd really appreciate that. What did you think of that art exhibit we saw this afternoon?

This response misses several points.

First, by calling attention to her position—that she believes eating animals is offensive—she *would* be ruining their fun, even if she claims she is not trying to do that. They know how easily a vegan changes the dynamics; that is why they can't ask her how her meal is. They have to be blocked about her vegetarianism—that is their survival strategy at the moment.

Second, no, they can't show a little respect for her. If they could have, they would have. That they haven't says they can't. It's really that simple. Asking for respect in this situation would not achieve anything. The bonding that is happening is directed from the top down, not from below up.

The third error in this approach is that it ignores the fact that many people are insensitive. They *do* tell anti-Semitic jokes in front of Jews, racist jokes in front of African Americans, sexist jokes in front of women. By using Jewishness as an example, she may offend someone who is Jewish and is there. They may not like the comparison. And it misses the point anyway. After all, the joking is part of their defense mechanism as blocked vegetarians.

Fourth, since she has so little to eat, she could quickly take control of the conversation by telling a long, involved joke or fascinating story. She would succeed in changing the subject, and would be remembered as the one with the interesting story. She doesn't need to tell them what she is doing ("I am going to get your—and my—mind off these poor lobsters"), she just does it.

The fact is, this isn't about her. It's about the company. Is she a team player or not? This is a loyalty test. Remember, two important characteristics of a loyalty test are that people act out of character in a controlled environment and the tests happen infrequently. This is exactly what transpired in this situation.

Even if what you are experiencing is a loyalty test, it does not mean you need to allow your deepest principles to be violated. Instead, develop survival skills for these times of testing. Prepare for them: at the restaurant leave the table and make your food arrangements; detach, meditate, even get ill, if need be, and excuse yourself early from the evening.

THE BUSINESS LUNCH

Business lunches are different. They are repetitive in their problems. Often, the problem is that meat eaters are going out to eat at restaurants that cannot or appear not to be able to accommodate you. The less power you have in a relationship, the more vulnerable your eating practices will be. Job-related duties require eating with meat eaters at some pretty disturbing places.

One person, who is now able to control this, makes sure that no business meetings occur over meals. After years of working under bosses who required her to attend business meetings where lots of meat was eaten, this immensely relieves the stress on her. "It seems like the coward's way out, but I got so tired of being made to feel like I was a 'problem' just for being different when really I was feeling guilty for not being *more* of a 'problem' and telling them my opinion!"

But this does not relieve the problem for those of you who are in a work environment in which there is little control. Draw upon all the precautions available as described in Chapter 11, "Grace at Work: Eating with Meat Eaters."

Here is how one person handled a demanding situation. A woman who worked as a biodecontamination specialist was a liaison with an animal health company that specialized in the poultry industry. The vegetarian headed off to Arkansas to meet some of the key players and important customers. After meeting in a hotel room, the eight of them went out to eat.

We went to a prime-rib buffet. My heart sank as I previewed the choices to come: meat, meat, and more meat, mashed potatoes slathered in gravy, vegetables swimming in butter. There was virtually not a single dish on the buffet that was entirely plant based. Then I noticed the salad bar—a separate area, and I knew I would find sustenance!

I took a huge plate and loaded it up with lettuce and other vegetables until it could not possibly hold anything else. I selected what I thought would strategically be the best place to sit at the large rectangular table we would all share—the first chair from the end—hoping that my food selections would be more obscure there. We were perhaps five minutes into the meal when the poultry farmer sitting directly across the table from me looked over at my plate. Then he looked up at me. I watched him quickly glance around the table in turn at everyone's plates before returning to look at me, then he said, "So what's the deal . . . are you a vegetarian or WHAT?!" I sat there for a moment dumbfounded. I hadn't anticipated such a direct confrontation based solely upon what my plate looked like. I knew that if I appeared to have any ethical basis for the selection of my food it would pretty much sabotage my new job. I looked around the table slowly at each of the men. All were significantly overweight with large protruding beer bellies. Then I looked at their plates—layer upon layer of dead flesh swimming in liquefied fats. A few overcooked vegetables peeked out from underneath yet even more fat. Then I spoke:

"Well, sort of . . . well, no, not really . . . but then I guess kind of . . . well, ever since my father's scare with heart disease, the whole family eats this way." Silence fell over the table. Most of the men looked down at their plates. Then one by one they spoke up.

"Yeah, my doctor says I've got to get my cholesterol down, too."

"My blood pressure is way too high."

"I'm supposed to be on a diet. . . . I shouldn't even be eating this stuff."

After nearly everyone had made such a confession, the conversation moved on. I was never again hassled about my eating, and I

learned an important lesson for survival in my new position. I never
called myself a vegetarian, but I spoke endlessly about fat and choles-
terol and conveyed that it was these things I was concerned about—as
a result of my father's experience.

Her choice, and it was very wise, was to avoid becoming a target. She needed to be seen as like them, not different from them. She avoided the word *vegetarian*. She did not let their worlds collide. This is what the business meal is, after all, supposedly an opportunity to consolidate business relationships. She did not feel that she sacrificed her vegetarian identity; she simply repackaged it, making it accessible.

Do not use business lunches to try to accomplish what even ordinary mixed meals cannot usually do—teaching about vegetarianism. Review the guidelines for talking with meat eaters and add this one: If my vegetarianism becomes an explicit issue, how does this further the purpose of this function? If there is no answer, then follow the advice for eating out and be prepared. If this feels as though you are being asked to violate an integral part of you, begin to identify other possible work environments that would not require this compromise.

COMPANY PERKS

You can be pretty sure that some company functions are going to either exclude you or offend you. One woman negotiated that she did not have to participate in company functions at such places if clients were not involved. But "in a lot of ways my vegan viewpoint made me an outsider in company affairs, and I missed out on many events that were arranged casually where I would not be invited because of my dietary choices." This might be holiday parties or casual staff get-togethers. At those events, spontaneous ideas and programs may be hatched. You will be aware of having been excluded.

If some problems recur because of business relationships, identify the pattern and ask: What can I do about it? What can be changed here?

Another company issue is holiday gifts. One woman wrote:

At my job, the Christmas gift from the company is a ham, turkey, and some sausage. I told the executive secretary (she handles the gift order-ing) that she could give mine to someone else, as I would just throw it away. . . . She looked at me as if I grew a third eye.

Yes, the gift is insensitive. But so was the vegetarian's response.

MEAT EATING LEADS TO VEGETARIANISM

A friend of mine, James, is a UPS truck driver. He tells me that at first his co-workers viewed him as strange because of his vegetar-ianism. Now, several years later, those same co-workers approach him for health information whenever they have an ailment or concern.

Think about it: the flow is in our direction. Meat eating leads to vegetarianism because of doctors' orders. Your co-workers may approach you tentatively for information. But they will do so only if they feel that you aren't judging them. When you start to relate to your colleagues, and they to you, in a humane way, your diet will actually open up the possibility of making connections. It just takes a lot of time and patience. Janice wrote of her experience working at an insurance company:

When I started working, my boss Pete ate McDonald's hamburgers with salt on them, doughnuts and coffee for breakfast; he smoked and had a nightly drink (one or two). One year later he was eating bran muffins with black coffee or water for breakfast, turkey sandwiches with water or juice for lunch, quit smoking, started jogging again, and cut most of his drinking. He didn't turn vegetarian, but he turned his bad habits out.

One vegan keeps fail-proof recipes in a stack in her office, to give to people who are curious. Inevitably the movement is from meat eat-ing to vegetarianism.

BUILDING A NEW TEAM

One can build a new team by trying to change the system or by changing jobs. For one vegan, change did occur, because she was able to articulate clearly her ethical stance:

> *We had a worldwide sales meeting that culminated in an awards dinner at a marine park. I told my boss that I would not be able to attend for ethical reasons. After questioning me closely, he reluctantly agreed that I could miss the dinner. He then came back to me a few days later and said that, after thinking carefully about the issue and talking to friends and family, he had determined that no company event in the future would be held in any place that had a likelihood of offending people in this way. Although he did not share my views, he believed them to be sincerely held and to be as strong a reason for consideration as those of any religious or ethnic group.*

Clearly, the boss was able to hear her, and was not using the meeting as a loyalty test. Another woman tried to change a very alienating environment:

> *I used to work at a Humane Society (who served chicken at balls and galas). I was one of a handful of vegetarians. On Meat Out day [a national drive for vegetarianism on the first day of spring], I did a presentation about going vegetarian. I couldn't understand how these people could take care of dogs and cats and then eat other animals. Many were receptive and gave up eating animals; however, I found a note on my desk (unsigned) asking me not to talk about vegetarian issues since some people ate meat and it made them uncomfortable.*

Eventually she had to ask herself, "Is this the team I want to be playing on?" All work involves some compromise, unless we are self-employed (in which case uncompromising positions may be self-destructive but at least are yours alone to deal with). You need to decide what your bottom line is. Does your job conflict with your belief system? If it does, you are going to be expending energy that is blocking your ethical position so that you can survive the atmosphere at work. At this point, we understand what happens to blocked energy. It leaks into other aspects of your life. It is also exhausting blocking it. Are you helping to arrange the financing for a chicken processing plant? Do you work in a health food store and have to stock the meat department? You might discover you have to change jobs. Clearly, if you become a vegetarian, you might not want to continue in an occupation such as butcher, meat packer, being a waiter in a steakhouse, a lobbyist for the cattle industry. Your job might be involved in some peripheral way with the meat industry, like the woman who found herself in Arkansas with a plateful of salad among her clients in the poultry industry.

If you are exhausted by having to balance the demands of your job with a changed consciousness about food and animals, see this as an opportunity to change more than your diet. This may be the opportunity you have been waiting for to try something new. You yourself might be blocked in developing a skill or have a secret dream. Perhaps you want to get more involved in the not-for-profit world. Turn to books such as *The Artist's Way, What Color Is Your Parachute?*, or *The Inner Art of Vegetarianism Workbook,* to help you access a deeper, more authentic self.

If you are happy in your job, and can negotiate the rapids of the meat-eating business world in which you find yourself, you might decide that volunteering with a health, environmental, vegetarian, or animal advocacy group meets the needs of this evolving authentic self.

To be on the job does not mean having to be on display, under attack, ganged up on, burnt out, or constantly alienated. If this is your situation, then you are being seriously deprived of the conditions for living with a sense of abundance. Honestly appraise what is working against your best self and find ways to work for, with, and on behalf of it.

13

Magician at Work: Cooking for Meat Eaters

Vegetarian chef! Isn't that an oxymoron?" my brother-in-law Bill asked when I had confessed that if I weren't a writer I would like to be a vegan chef. Many meat eaters hold this opinion. Oh sure, they'd give up meat . . . if the food we offered tasted good. The problem, they say, is that vegetarian food is tasteless, textureless.

I knew he said those words ironically, as he sat there devouring my grilled sourdough biscuits and nutty cabbage salad. That evening, as I was preparing them, and some tofu "steaks," my sister Nancy came up to me and declared, "I know what you are doing. You are going to convert us just by good taste alone." We had not seen each other for a year, and this was our first meal together. She was right; why not cut through all the anxieties and defenses and simply let people eat good, tasty food lovingly prepared? What better gift from our lives to theirs can be given?

We are magicians. "Watch my left hand," we say as we do the magic with our right hand. This is what we are doing with our cooking. What's my right hand doing? Preparing this vegetarian food so that my left hand can offer it to you. You don't have to know what my right hand is doing. You don't have to be reminded of the fact that this is vegetarian food. Instead, we make magic happen.

And when it happens once, we want to make it happen again and again. Perhaps, if you are like me, you go from being an uninspired cook to a demon cook. The alchemical process of changing—not just changing ourselves but changing foods into delectable dishes—repeatedly draws us back again. That is why I found myself telling my sister of my deep physical need to cook. "I can't explain it or understand it." I shrug. "I want to be in the kitchen preparing food, handling vegetables and fruits, participating in the alchemy of mixing together ingredients and creating a delectable meal."

And that is why, on the hottest day of a very hot summer, I am in my parents' kitchen, standing before the sink, washing sweet potatoes; in front of the stove, toasting walnuts; at the chopping block, slicing tomatoes, chopping up fresh rosemary, mincing garlic; and at the food processor with my fourteen-year-old son creating a vegan pesto. My sister has said, "Why don't you prepare the meal for Saturday night?" Fifteen people will be there. I make Caribbean sweet potato salad, tofu steaks (marinated in red wine vinegar, olive oil, and soy sauce), rosemary sourdough bread, salad with raspberry vinaigrette, a tomato tart, angel hair with pesto, and a gingered fruit crisp with peaches, nectarines, blueberries, and blackberries. We stop to pick up some corn on the cob and accompany the farmer into the field as she picks the corn. As she examines the corn, she explains to us that she feels for plumpness in the kernels and looks at the hair on the top of the corn to determine if it is ready to be picked.

It has been so hot that the insects are eating the blueberries for the water. It is so hot that I think, "How could I have agreed to cook today of all days?" But then, over supper, the reason is clear. Magic is happening. I realize with a thrill, everyone is enjoying this food! No one has noticed that anything is missing. That is because nothing is missing! They feel comfortable. Everyone feels casual, relaxed. Even my father, a man who I thought still believed there should be meat at a meal, is instead conversing about the pesto, taking on the role of woeful but secretly proud father: "If I don't plant two different kinds of basil, *she* [gesturing in my direction] won't come home in the summer!"

The foods came together to touch all the senses: the beauty of the tomatoes and basil sitting in a puff pastry shell, the smell of the fresh pesto, the fruit crisp with ginger infusing the fruit.

And in this feast, when the meal is successful and they love the food, like any magician, I am pleased with my sleight of hand. No one needs to know the particulars of what has happened. We give something from our lives to enhance theirs, something that we have created out of love. Love of good food, well prepared, is contagious.

We have the greatest gift of all: we know the joy of food lovingly prepared that is humane. This is the key to living among meat eaters. Find in yourself a way to share it. Cooking is one way to negotiate difficult relationships, one way that says, "I love you. Let me share this with you."

Meat eaters are free to enter a loving, nonjudgmental space. By presenting good food, we let them know that we are not judging them and we give them the space not to judge themselves. They can simply be. Then they can experience grace. And they may realize this might be a place to which they wish to return because they will associate it with positive emotions—of hunger satisfied and guilt released. Here, eating our food, they are not blocked vegetarians. They are experiencing vegetarianism directly.

SHOW, DON'T TELL

Show, don't tell. Why? Good food assuages inchoate feelings and fears. Meat eaters know what they are giving up. They don't yet know what they are getting in return. The unknown is scary. They may fear being a vegetarian.

The Central Fears That Meat Eaters Have Concerning a Vegetarian Meal

1. That they'll be hungry. They may truly feel anxiety because they think they will not be full without meat.
2. The demands of change: everything will be different, there will be nothing familiar and they think they need to stick with the familiar. (Remember, they may be neophobes!)

3. That you're trying to change them.

4. Loss of variety. That vegetarian food is bland and boring.

5. That vegetarian food *isn't* bland and boring. Then they won't have an excuse.

6. That they *won't* miss the meat.

7. That being a vegetarian is difficult.

8. That being a vegetarian *isn't* difficult.

9. A fear about friends/peers—what will I feed them?

Your meal is doing more than serving them nutritious calories; it can also help to calm their fears about what the absence of meat entails. Or what your intentions are.

Meat eaters often think, "What will I replace meat with?" This focuses energy on perpetuating the idea of its absence. We simply show them this is not a problem. Or, meat eaters think, "I'll replace meat with tofu and I don't want to do that!" The fear of tofu is a special problem.

Tofu-Phobia

Some nonvegetarians have a deep, abiding, irrational fear of tofu. They are tofu-phobes. Tofu represents vegetarianism to them. Their greatest fear is that they will have to eat tofu. When one tofu-phobe I know is attending vegetarian functions, he says, "I hope there is something edible there, something that you don't have to think about whether it's something you use for home repair or apparel."

Tofu-phobes are guilty of (false) syllogistic thinking:

Tofu is yucky.

Vegetarians eat tofu.

Vegetarianism is yucky.

One vegan friend of mine believes that people need to feel their jaws moving or else they feel they haven't eaten. This may be why tofu is disliked so intensely. Liberation from tofu-phobia can occur in one of two ways: They are exposed to tofu that is tasty and delicious, or they discover that vegetarianism does not require tofu.

One friend, Sarah, told of preparing a meal for her family:

> *I cooked a meal for my family—portobello mushrooms with noodles and marinara. I didn't think of it as making a vegetarian meal, I just thought of it as proving I could cook. But my dad said, "If vegetarians eat like this, I could do that. I thought it was all salad and tofu."*

We have more variety in our diets after becoming vegetarians than before. Though we may tell them so, it can be hard for meat eaters to comprehend this. But we can show them. A vegetarian law student who cooked feasts every weekend, reported to me, "When people ask me what I eat, I tell them. I run off a list of things, then I invite them over to my next big dinner."

All that is required for meat eaters to be open to vegetarianism is for them to eat vegetarian foods in a nonthreatening atmosphere. Meat eaters are filled with beliefs about meat, about eating, about vegetarianism. When we act in such a way as to confirm their beliefs about vegetarianism, we simply fill them further. The more they are filled with meat eating and their beliefs, the less space they have to experience vegetarianism. That is why we show, don't tell.

Meat eaters have to believe in their own possibility for being vegetarian rather than someone else's possibility. Instead of having to answer the frequently posed question "Don't you miss meat?" we let them experience that they had a vegan meal and *they* didn't miss the meat. Until they have that experience, they are most likely eating the menu, not the meal.

EATING THE MENU, NOT THE MEAL

Philosopher and interpreter of Eastern religions Alan Watts observed that people eat the menu rather than the meal. That is, people eat the *idea* of what they are eating, not the *reality* of it. How do we know this? They unintentionally reveal it. A friend's husband was an adamant meat eater. Her sister was vegetarian. At a holiday dinner, the husband was happily eating a vegetarian lasagna and praising its taste. He did not know that what he was enjoying was a TVP lasagna. Suddenly he looked around the table. His *vegetarian* sister-in-law was eating the lasagna, too! He was shocked. "Hey, wait a minute, what's in this?" he demanded. As long as he thought he was eating his traditional lasagna, he was happy. The food did not change—only his awareness did.

A meat eater discovers he is eating the same food as a vegetarian. His traditional view was "How good can it be if a vegetarian is eating it?" but this time, he knows otherwise. It is good. He *was* enjoying it. This is the magician at work—allowing a nonvegetarian to experience life as a vegetarian. What the meat eater discovers is that such a life does not involve constant self-consciousness nor the giving up of tasty food. We have to speak to the feeling, tasting, sensing, smelling, looking part of them with our food rather than telling them anything. We can't tell them the menu; we simply have to share the meal.

At our wedding reception, the main course was walnut balls in a béchamel sauce. Everyone was convinced it was meat and they thought I had capitulated. "Oh, Carol has given in. And aren't these the most delicious meatballs!" They enjoyed those walnut balls so much! This was a profound experience for me. They were holding on to the menu. Their stomachs didn't know the difference; but as long as their minds were so convinced, it didn't matter what was going into their stomachs.

How to Handle Menu-Eating Guests

Miss Manners once got a long letter from some vegetarians about how to refuse meat being offered to them. Rightly, she advised, say "No thanks" and leave it at that. The letter also raised another problem: guests who bring meat to eat when they are houseguests of a vegetarian. Curiously, Miss Manners did not respond to this section of the letter. What should Miss Manners have answered when she heard about a weekend guest who brought bacon to go with his eggs and brought cold cuts for lunch? She should have said:

Dear Gentle Veggie:

You do not have to accept this practice. This houseguest has either had too little or too much exposure to vegetarianism—either not understanding it at all or misunderstanding it all too well. He sounds like a meat eater who thinks, "I must defend myself against their vegetarianism. I don't want to know what a weekend without meat is like. I don't want to know it is possible. I want to continue believing that it is impossible." He is trying to establish control in a situation where he feels loss of control. As one vegetarian friend, Francine, observes: "If your guests comment on the fact that meat is missing, your problem is rude guests, not a bad menu." That is your houseguest's main problem—not meat eating but rudeness.

Treat his actions as rudeness. You can say, "Oh, David, I'm sorry you didn't realize that cooking meat in our house just isn't acceptable. We know you regret causing us consternation. We'll freeze this for you so you can take it with you." And then show him the alternatives to these foods.

If David says, "This dish would be perfect if it had some meat in it," you can say: "When you make it you can put it in." End of discussion.

Who's Eating My Food?

Another vegetarian had the opposite problem. He lived with meat eaters who were eating the meal, *his* meal, not the menu, *their* menu. And they weren't being very honest about their choices. I'll let him explain it:

I am a vegan who lives with a family of meat eaters. Since I live with meat eaters I often have to get my own foods. There have been occasions where the meat-eating family members have taken my foods and finished them without asking me. As a vegan, I encourage people to substitute vegan foods for nonvegan ones in the hope that they will switch to using vegan products. But when foods that were meant for you, because there is nothing else that you will eat in a house with meat eaters, were consumed without your knowledge, I think it is inconsiderate on the part of your housemates or family members.

Should we just forget about it or tell them to be more considerate? But how do you do it without giving them the impression that you are some selfish vegan? If I were a rich vegan, I would simply buy more vegan foods for everyone in the family. But if you are a vegan like me, struggling to make ends meet, it will bother you if this will become a problem, and you will soon start worrying about your food experiences if you decide to keep quiet about it. Especially when they have confirmed that they have no intention of even considering trying veganism or vegetarianism.

I would advise him:

Dear Gentle Veggie:

Your problem is that you live with a dishonest family. Because they can't be honest with themselves about their interest in and enjoyment of your food, they prefer to steal it from you. They do not want to bring to consciousness their own interest in your food. They want to be able to eat your food without dealing with its implications in their lives. They may also be lazy.

How do you avoid having them think "you are some selfish vegan"? You do it like this: know your bottom line and protect it. They are abusing you and presuming upon your niceness. They assume you will let them continue to be selfish. You did not move in with the idea of subsidizing their food budget. It is perfectly okay to say, "Look, I know you say you aren't interested in my food, but you are doing something different. You are eating it. Let me fix a meal a week for the household, and those leftovers will be available to everyone. Or, before I go shopping for myself, I will announce what

I plan to make. If you think you want some, let me know. I will pro-rate the cost of the food." You could also offer to do the shopping for the household. Together create a list. Notice what vegan items they tend to take most frequently and after the list is made, add these to the list. The key here is to make these foods available without making it obvious.

Some vegans might confront their housemates. You clearly are not comfortable with this. The most effective choice, if it is at all possible, is moving. No matter what their food choices are, you are living with people who are not above lying and stealing. This is not a conducive environment for anyone—especially one who ends up undernourished because of them!

His housemates were eating his meal, not their menu. *This* is the power of delicious vegan food.

STAGES OF COOKING FOR MEAT EATERS

Everyone is a potential vegetarian. In preparing vegetarian meals for meat eaters, we help them experience their own relationship with vegetarianism.

Stage 1: Nonchalance and Familiarity

My friend Karen Davis, founder of United Poultry Concerns, says that what people love to eat is food that is "crispy, crunchy, chewy, oily, spicy." Another friend says that people are used to salty, sweet, rich, and buttery things. We need to appeal to their palate by making food colorful and textured. Unless you have a tried-and-true tofu recipe or one that thoroughly disguises it, at this stage avoid cooking with tofu. Take familiar foods and cook with them in a different way. This shows them that vegetarianism/veganism isn't all "tofu." You need to allay their fear of scarcity.

One vegan cook, Annette, explains why staying with the familiar is her first choice:

> It certainly made my transition easier. I choose something simple. In our fast-paced society, it seems doomed to failure to prepare a complicated vegetarian meal for a meat eater in hopes that after they say, "I didn't miss the meat," they'll want to cook it themselves. I make sure I send via the mail, though, recipes and handy tips for those who are trying vegetarianism/veganism. Plus, this keeps the communication lines open. And that I care about them and their success and if they become frustrated or whatever, they can call.

"Know thy guest." As Virginia and Mark Messina explain in their book *The Vegetarian Way,* "Your friends who are world travelers and lovers of new experiences will be thrilled to try a spicy vegetable curry or a savory Indonesian tempeh stew. But when Uncle Dave, who has never eaten a meatless meal in his life, comes for dinner, it's a good idea to put away the sprouts, sea vegetables, and sesame tahini." Their bottom line: "Know when to be exotic and when to be basic in your meal planning. . . . Be elegant rather than earthy."

Tips for This Stage of Cooking

- Use more fat—"That's one of the addictive ingredients in animal foods," says Billy Ray Boyd, author of *For the Vegetarian in You.*
- Avoid that which could be seen as strange.
- Go ethnic—either your ethnic tradition, or one that is already familiar to your guest.
- Don't name the ingredients until their suspicions are down.
- Prepare familiar foods with new flavors. You might roast cashews and toss them into a salad.

- Everyone loves soup. Everyone loves stews. And maybe even chili.
- Pasta, pasta, pasta.
- Do not try to compensate for a lack of meat.
- Use more salt.
- Cut the vegetables in large pieces, so they don't get all mashed into a stew (unless a stew is your goal!). This way the eye has something to focus on. Some people fear foods that are all mixed up together.
- Flavor and balance can come from vinegars (from mild rice vinegar to very acidic sherry vinegar). If a soup tastes as though it needs salt, it might actually need acid (vinegar, a squeeze of lemon or lime juice, or some wine).
- Reorder the plate. Anticipate that there is anxiety about what will replace meat and whether there will be a gaping hole. Create main courses that announce themselves and have an attention-grabbing appearance. Create a crepe cake: stacked and impressive. Create main-course cobblers.
- Stuff favorite vegetables or vegetable mixtures such as rata-touille into phyllo or puff pastry or make them into tarts. These convey a sense of abundance.
- Use sauces to give food "body." See Joanne Stepaniak's *The Saucy Vegetarian* for endless ideas.

Stage 2: Kitchen Magic

In this stage of cooking, bring meat eaters into the kitchen so that they can see how easy vegetarian food is to prepare. Be sure to have tried-and-true recipes. Now you can introduce tofu and other alternatives.

Learn from fancy restaurants: name all the vegetables dishes you serve. Perhaps it is a hangover from commands to "eat *your* vegetables" or from cooks trained in the old way—"Place vegetables in boiling water, remove twenty minutes later and serve"—but many meat eaters have no faith in vegetables. You aren't serving just vegetables but "roast

vegetables with fennel seeds and garlic with a balsamic vinegar bath."
This may capture someone's attention and their taste buds, too.

Stage 3: Even the Unfamiliar Can Be Familiar

Because change can be scary, one answer is showing meat eaters that
they really don't have to change—well, not much. For those who seem
truly interested, introduce them to foods that help wean them from
meat eating (tofu dogs, seitan, veggie burgers, TVP). Introduce them to
the approach a vegetarian has to everyday cooking.

EVERYDAY COOKING
FOR MEAT EATERS

You may live in a household of meat eaters. How do you handle
your cooking responsibilities?

- Identify your household's ten basic meals. Which ones are
  already vegetarian? Macaroni and cheese? Baked potatoes?
  Soups? Which ones can become vegetarian? In place of the
  meat and dairy, make substitutions: spaghetti and meatballs
  can become spaghetti in a mushroom sauce, spaghetti with
  tofu balls, spaghetti with TVP.
- Develop new recipes using their favorite vegetarian food as
  a base. For instance, if it is the perennial family favorite, pasta,
  you can make spaghetti primavera, spaghetti marinara, Asian
  noodles. You can make grilled pizzas, veggie pizzas, pesto
  pizzas.
- Identify what your household has traditionally rejected.
  Now is not the time to start working with it. If they have
  always hated squash, don't offer them a stuffed squash for
  their main course.

- Create mix-and-match meals. Make your own burritos, with choices of beans, rice, lettuce, salsa, tomatoes, mushrooms, tofu or TVP, corn, peppers, or whatever you prefer.

- Make enough food to freeze some for a night when someone else is cooking the meal so that they can have meat. This way you have something to eat and can stay out of the kitchen.

- Make a commitment to add a new vegetable or cooking technique every week/two weeks/month. Serve the new food with ones that are already accepted.

- Go ethnic. Many cuisines use meat as a condiment, not as a main course. Select dishes that could have meat added to them if the diners so desired (stir-fries, curries, Middle Eastern platters). Give the household the choice to prepare something for themselves to go with the main dish that you are preparing.

DON'T CALL ATTENTION TO THE MEAL'S VEGETARIANISM

I have recommended not talking about vegetarianism in the presence of meat. This recommendation also applies to a complete vegan meal: keep out of the way of the food. You can't talk a vegan meal. It has to be experienced. This recommendation arises from one final Adams maxim: *"Nonvegetarians are perfectly happy eating a vegan meal, as long as they are not aware they are doing so."* Don't take attention away from the food. Let the food speak. What matters is the joy of the time together and the creative meal being offered. In talking, less is more; in cooking, more is more. Less talking, more time and space to experience a meal. You are saying: Here I am. Here is my delicious food. Let me share it.

I am not advising that you do this in a deliberately sneaky way, a sort of "I'll show them!" approach. Just as you do not want people to surprise you with ingredients you don't wish to eat, so, too, you do not want to act this way toward others. But preparing and serving food in a relaxed way, in which the contents of the meal unfold in the serving, neither hiding nor proclaiming, is an approach that can put people at ease.

People's relationship to food when they are eating has to be casual, relaxed, no tension. I don't want to lecture. And they don't want to hear a lecture. That would change the focus from food to ideas. To lecture about vegetarianism requires pulling from a different part of the brain to explain it. You want to relax, and so do they.

When you don't talk about it, their guard isn't up. They may feel suspicious of vegetarians: "What are you trying to put over on me?" And feeling suspicious, they wish to establish that they are the ones who will decide: "I will not be controlled or manipulated by someone else!"

People think, "It can't be done. You can't have pesto without Parmesan cheese. It won't taste right." Don't tell them before you serve them that in fact you have left the Parmesan cheese out. Wait. Then there is no need to convince with words because they themselves have experienced it.

Everyone enjoys pleasant surprises. However, in most cases, people don't want to know in advance that they are being surprised. They don't like knowing that you know something they don't or that you are experimenting on them or forcing them to eat something. Let the meal speak for itself. Don't talk about it because they will be suspicious of your motives for serving them—they fear that you want to convert them. You need to make clear that you want to share with them, not convert them. If they are suspicious of your intentions, this self-consciousness will interfere with the joy the food should and can impart. They may feel that they have been "forced" to eat a vegetarian meal.

Let the vegetarian food work at a nonverbal level. Let it be comforting, filling. If you talk about it, people may feel, "Isn't it enough I'm eating it? Do I also have to think about it?"

Vegetarians who stop showing and start sharing, who stop talking about meat eating and simply cook for meat eaters from their place of contentment, report a change in people around themselves when they change. When they have emptied themselves of expectations and frustrations with the meat eaters in their lives, they feel freedom and acceptance and offer a welcoming spirit; they embrace people where they are. And suddenly, all around them, people are becoming vegans. When they let go of expectations and reactions, they give people the space to find their own relationship. Our freedom from expectations brings about their freedom to decide their own relationship to food. They can be more open, because we have given them that space.

After all, they have to experience not *our* experience of the feeling of abundance we get from our food, but *their* own feeling of abundance that can come from eating this food. The minute they are conscious that they aren't eating meat, they may not feel abundance, because that feeling has always accompanied the sense that "I can choose whatever food I want and no one is going to tell me otherwise." They may lose that feeling if they see you as choosing their food, not themselves.

Most important, when the meal is unlabeled and yet all can eat, the meat eater–vegetarian dualism that the meat eater blames you for creating has been banished. Awareness isn't about choices we have made in the past, but about simply experiencing this good meal. We say to them very calmly, through the food we prepare, "My diet can incorporate you in many ways that are unthreatening."

People think, "I can't be fooled. I know how they are doing this magic trick." But they can be fooled and they may not understand the magic trick. "Fooling them" is actually not your intention; it is your only way to get around their tendency to eat the menu instead of the meal. And when you have succeeded, don't rub it in that you have "fooled" them. Let them experience the surprise and process this information themselves. This is part of the incubation process that each person needs to become unblocked.

THE ALCHEMY OF A MEAL

Alchemy is the seemingly magical power of changing one substance into another. The vegetarian meal's alchemy occurs not in the cooking but in the serving of what has been prepared. Almost magically, the enjoyment of this great vegetarian food by meat eaters creates a feeling of joy within us, the vegetarians, and, to their surprise, within them. People enjoy this food. That is the biggest aspect of vegetarianism that is constantly denied. Yes, there are all the jokes about tofu, and all the complaints from papers like the *New York Times* to the local paper about veggie burgers or "not dogs" or some other clearly identified "vegetarian" food. But when people sit down to eat a vegetarian meal, delights can abound:

My roommate absolutely refused to eat anything that I made once I became a vegetarian. Maybe some vegetables but definitely no tofu or TVP. I made TVP chili one night. I left some on the table and my roommate told me how good it smelled. I offered him some. "Is there TVP in it?" Yes, I answered. Then, "Uhhhh, no." Anyway, I had to do some computer work and left the dish on the table. Then my roommate came up to me by the computer and asked if I had wanted any of the rest of the chili. Why? He had finished the whole thing, which was at least two or three servings. He said it was so good.

An example like this proves my point that meat eaters' greatest fear may be that they in fact do not miss the meat. Eating our food, they discover it is true. They don't miss the meat. Their question becomes, Given that they can enjoy vegetarian food, now how do they handle their blockedness? But that is not our concern, it is theirs. Our concern is to create good foods that suspicious, doubting meat eaters devour. This is hospitality. Host and guest both experience freedom in relationship with each other; they are free to express themselves and discover new aspects of themselves and their relationship. The food unites us; it doesn't separate us.

Alchemy eliminates the awareness that there is a gestalt shift. What has appeared to be divisive is transcended by bringing the meat eaters into our meals. They discover that a vegetarian does not necessarily provoke defensiveness. Here, in this space, we have all returned to being simply eaters. There are no "meat eaters." There are no "vegetarians."

There are people sitting around a table sharing food and talk. Here taste, touch, and smell relax us.

People want food to unite them. Vegetarians appear to threaten this unity. We have to help people experience that unity. Creating a vegetarian meal without labeling it such allows a meat eater to be pulled into the flow, to experience a connection with us without it being labeled. In Chapter 2, I discussed the way vegetarianism automatically creates a dualism, especially from the meat eater's perspective. But in a good meal enjoyed by everyone, without labels, there is communion, coming together, not being broken apart. The process grounds the mind within the body, allowing the discovery that this food is enjoyable. Later, at a time when the minds of meat eaters wander back to the meal, they will think: "Carol created that meal. That was a tasty meal. Carol doesn't eat meat or dairy products. . . . That meal didn't have any meat or dairy products. . . . I ate a delicious meal that didn't have any meat or dairy products. . . . I *enjoyed* a meal that didn't have meat or dairy products." In this moment of discovery, that evening or later, in reverie, the meat eater realizes that he or she experienced vegetarianism without any defensiveness. This grants them the freedom of discovery and reflection. This is their own alchemical process—the discovery that a vegetarian chef is not an oxymoron. And the next day, they ask this magician for the leftovers.

14

Being the Mover, Not the Moved

Talking to Charles Stahler of the Vegetarian Resource Group, I said to him, "I'm trying to finish my book *Living Among Meat Eaters.*" He laughed and said, "You can either write your book or live among meat eaters, but you can't do both." It was funny because in some ways it is true. The meat-eating world can take a lot of your energy!

But when you see yourself as living among blocked vegetarians, you can transform any interaction. Once you realize they are blocked, you are aware of what prompts their interactions with you. They sense a connection they can't make; we are enabled to continue to make connections we desire to make. You become the mover instead of the moved.

It is true that for nearly ten years I have been trying to write this book. It took me longer than I thought it would to write it because I had to become the person who could write this book. That may sound strange, but to me, now, it is self-evident. When I began this book I was angry with meat eaters. That anger was short-circuiting my own thought processes. In my relationships, I was being moved rather than being the mover.

Because of the growth of vegetarianism, meat eaters interact with vegetarians more frequently than before. This brings their blockedness to consciousness more frequently. It creates a state of rawness in which the status quo is battling more furiously to maintain itself. This may explain why there are more tensions being experienced right now. Will we be the movers or the moved?

Three things happened that helped me become the "mover" rather than the "moved." I began keeping a more detailed journal. In doing this, I put myself and my interactions under a microscope. Vegetarian–meat eater issues would appear in it. But so would my own personal needs and quirks. Surprise! As any journal keeper knows, issues reappear. And when they reappear and reappear, one suddenly thinks, "What is *this* issue? Why is it *still* recurring?" Then, if growth is to happen, you inquire of yourself, "What's the next step?" As a writer, I thought, "There is a pattern to these interactions!" The pattern is the systemic issues this book addresses. My own experience is augmented by more than two hundred surveys that were returned to me from vegetarians about their experiences living among meat eaters. The patterns I found in my own life appeared in these surveys, too.

In my own path toward a systemic understanding, another important ingredient was making a commitment to meditate. As a theorist, I spend a lot of time with my mind and its thoughts. But this can be a trap. The mind has a way of limiting our experience of our own selves and our reality. Meditation helps me recognize that neither my thoughts nor my feelings constitute "me." I can observe these thoughts or feelings rather than be trapped by them. Achieving this distance from my own experience was extremely helpful. I stopped being moved.

Finally, I decided to take my life as a vegan more seriously. This involved several things. First, I had to recognize that no one could meet my needs but myself. Once I understood that, I began researching vegan cooking techniques and accumulating wonderful recipes, many of which I will share with you in the final chapter of this book. I realized that one of my responsibilities is to share this wonderful life with others.

What is gained by viewing meat eaters as blocked vegetarians? We gain an approach for difficult situations. We are able to restore to meat eaters the humanity their own actions sometimes deny. We can view them in a more positive, empathetic light because even their rudest and most frustrating actions are signs of their potential.

When we view meat eaters as blocked vegetarians, we learn from every interaction, especially the negative ones.

Meat eaters may be surprised that their responses are so transparent or so predictable. They may think their reactions are uniquely theirs, their arguments signs of their creativity, their humor revealing a quick wit. But we know better. They represent the responses of a class of people.

Viewing meat eaters as blocked vegetarians also gives us a place to stand, and a fulcrum. We truly are the mover rather than the moved. We are inviting them to us, not trying to conform to their agenda. In addition, we are optimistic: we believe in the possibility of change. We did it. Craven we may once have been, but we overcame our fears and cowardice. That is why we can believe in change for others: we were once there.

So, *is* every meat eater a blocked vegetarian? *Is* every meat-eater-related action a defense against vegetarianism?

Well, yes and no.

Yes, because as the aphorism goes, "If it walks like a duck and quacks like a duck, it is a duck." So, too, with meat eaters. I hear a lot of quacking; I see a lot of waddling.

But, maybe I'm wrong. Maybe meat eaters *aren't* blocked vegetarians. Still, any interaction can be transformed by approaching them as though they are blocked vegetarians. It enables us to interact with them without in any way trying to defend our vegetarianism. What is there to defend? Absolutely nothing. By becoming the mover instead of the moved, we find peace and speak from this place. The world becomes a place that is a sign not of meat eating's strength, but of its weaknesses. Just look at the disturbances we relatively few vegetarians cause a meat-eating majority!

You can make it into a game. You can ask of anything "What does this tell me about vegetarianism?" Consider *Jurassic Park*. What does that incredible blockbuster of a movie tell us about vegetarianism? That meat eaters harbor a fear that someone will do to them exactly what they are doing to the animals they eat: kill them and devour them. In *Jaws,* the fear of being treated like meat is prominent. And *Jurassic Park* adds a neat little twist to remind us of this theme: everyone is saved by the only vegetarian in the group—the adolescent girl.

What about another blockbuster of the 1990s? The movie *Titanic* hangs its story on an elderly woman who recaptures for an audience eighty years later the life and blood of the experience of the sinking of that great ship. For her age, Rose is quick-witted and agile. A woman about seventeen when the *Titanic* sank, she is a spry 101 when she narrates the story. Without her the movie would lose its narrative frame. Was the director, James Cameron, stretching reality in creating the fictional Rose? Actually Cameron based Rose on a neighbor of his, Beatrice Wood, a potter *and* a vegetarian. The story could be told by an elderly woman because Cameron had the model of a healthy and happy vegetarian centenarian before him.

Once you become the mover rather than the moved, you can make a great game of looking for the hidden vegetarian dynamic that propels a story (or an individual) from within. Indeed, one could do a vegetarian history of culture—from the great Asian religions that have their roots in the doctrine of *ahimsā,* nonharming, and advocate vegetarianism, to many of the creative geniuses of the Western world—da Vinci, Michelango, Thoreau. And anyone with a little time on their hands could do a fascinating study of the meat-eating anxieties expressed by cartoonists in the *New Yorker.* Lobsters eating lobstermen, cows who don't trust either presidential candidate because they are both carnivores, a fortune teller crying in a November issue, as she tells a turkey of her future. One cartoon was called "The Birth of a Vegetarian." In it, a man in a restaurant is about to take a bite of his steak when the steak says, "Moo." In that *New Yorker* cartoon the gestalt shift itself is captured: the moo from the steak reveals the life (and death) of an animal.

In *The Sexual Politics of Meat* I quoted Joseph Campbell, who observed that in cultures dependent on animal flesh, "the paramount object of experience is the beast. Killed and slaughtered it yields to people its flesh to become our substance, teeth to become our ornaments, hides for clothing and tents, sinews for ropes, bones for tools. The animal life is translated into human life entirely, through the medium of death, slaughter, and the arts of cooking, tanning, sewing." What else is Campbell saying but that a meat-eating world organizes itself around death? In fact, a meat-eating world does organize itself around death. Before the 9 billion land animals are killed, most of them are deadened to life by the factory farm system of managing animals. Our culture also organizes itself around death in the health care system. An average of $48,756 is spent on the last year of an individual's life. (How much do most of us spend in a given year?) Only recently has prevention begun to be emphasized rather than maintenance. And leading the change in emphasis is the vegetarian-based preventive program of Dr. Dean Ornish.

Campbell says that a plant-based world organizes itself around life. The plant world supplies "the food, clothing and shelter of people since time out of mind, but also our model of the wonder of life—in its cycle of growth and decay, blossom and seed, wherein death and life appear as transformations of a single, superordinated, indestructible force." Through the process of change the vegetarian does see the wonder of life—our own, if we become vegetarians for health reasons; the planet's, if we become vegetarians for environmental reasons; and the animals', if we become vegetarians for ethical reasons. The ability to step back from the culture of death and its manifestation at meals has nurtured something inside of the vegetarian that has been deadened in the meat eater. What keeps the meat eater blocked—the fears we discussed earlier—keeps unawakened, untouched, that part of the meat eater that could learn to deal with those fears. Because the vegetarian has dealt with death, at least this aspect of death, something has become alive in the vegetarian.

Living among meat eaters, we cannot lose this sense of life.

And we can look for signs of it in the culture at large—when vegetarianism leaks into cultural territory, so too does life. Rose, after all, is remarkable because she is still so vitally alive to tell the story. The twelve-year-old computer whiz in *Jurassic Park,* the vegetarian anchor in a carnivorous world, figures out how to use the computer to keep the carnivores out and so controls the mechanics of protecting human life.

Of all the correspondence I received over the years about living among meat eaters, one comment seemed especially poignant. One letter writer said, "Sometimes I feel like living without meat eaters around." Yes, interactions with them can be frustrating, depressing, or simply just tedious. They often kill off the possibility of relationships with them. Someday, though, maybe, just maybe, they will become unblocked vegetarians. Then we will all be able to live without meat eaters around. They will have joined us on the other side of the gestalt shift. Seeing them now as potential vegetarians we give this possibility— and so much more—life.

15

Recipes for Yourself and Others

When I was in my early twenties, I did not know how to handle a pepper. Now the words "roasted red pepper" trip effortlessly off my tongue. Not only do I handle, I roast! Vegetarianism is the main reason for this transformation. First, I had to learn how to cook. Then I wanted to know more, so much more that I now have over three hundred vegetarian cookbooks! Now I enjoy the process of learning and cooking. They are acts of renewal.

The following recipes are drawn from my experiences as a vegetarian cook for more than two decades. I have held on to some early vegetarian favorites and adapted them when I became a vegan. I have drawn upon regular cookbooks, vegetarian cookbooks, and vegan cookbooks.

Many of your favorite recipes can be easily veganized—transformed to a more humane but equally delicious dish. Whether this involves substituting a nondairy milk—soy, rice, or nut—for cow's milk, egg substitutes such as Ener-G Egg Replacer, tofu, a banana, or a flaxseed "slurry" for eggs in baked goods (¼ cup of flaxseeds blended for a couple of minutes in a dry blender, then add ¾ cup water. Blend and the result is a viscous, humane, and healthy equivalent of 3 eggs), or discovering ways of suggesting the taste of cheese without depending on dairy products— veganizing a recipe is an opportunity to learn about your own skills, your own creativity. (Examples of such transformation are, for instance, the béchamel sauce on page 244 or the comforting spinach soup on page 260.)

The goal is not just veganizing a recipe but personalizing it. If you like more cinnamon than the recipe calls for, fine! Add it. If you don't like onions, you can usually leave them out. Are you allergic to soy products? Learn about seitan. All recipes have a degree of flexibility, as most good cooks would acknowledge. There should be no tyranny of the recipe itself over you, the cook. Recipes are opportunities for exploration. Welcome them as an invitation to explore the connections among foods.

In working with recipes, I have often adapted ones from recipe books that I have enjoyed using. But, as you yourself will find, recipes—even these in this book—need to be "tweaked." I have changed quantities, veganized recipes, added or subtracted ingredients, altered the process of preparation, compared three or four similar recipes from different cookbooks—all in service of my desire for something that feels abundant and welcoming. You should assume this same methodology of transformation for these and any recipes you work with.

In our house, the arrangement that we have made for cooking is to follow the recipe the first time and then one may creatively alter it. We all comment on the recipe and whether it worked or not. Then I write notes on the pages of the recipe: the date, and the consensus of those who have eaten it. "Needs more [x]," I will write. Or, "Omit [y]." Some recipes are clearly "rejects" and I keep a folder of rejects to remind me of what has not worked. The highest achievement of a recipe is simply to have "tasty" written by its title. That means we all enjoyed this recipe and would be happy eating it again. The recipes that follow are mainly those that have been labeled "tasty."

Recipes included here are recipes that, to me, express abundance. In cooking for yourself and others, it is important to know what you experience as expressing abundance. I have noticed for myself that foods inside of other foods (turnovers, cobblers, and pies, for instance) convey a feeling of luxury. This says "abundance." You might not feel that way. You might, like my sons, like bulk. They need a different sort of abundance than I do. For them, the answer is pasta, pasta, pasta. Notice what excites you as you prepare food and what pleases you when you sit down to eat.

I happen to love tofu and am never happy if I go too many meals without tofu. You will find tofu overrepresented in these recipes; and seitan and tempeh underrepresented.

Rather than trying to replace the fat or texture of meat, I ask myself, What will convey abundance and joy? For me, besides fruit, it's mushrooms. Something about mushrooms generates a deep sense of peace. Notice your desires for certain foods, and how you respond to restaurant menus that list gourmet vegetarian items. Re-create the foods that interest you at home. If you enjoy cooking, page through your cookbook collection and find ways to adapt favorite recipes to your needs. My hope is that the recipes following will serve as inspiration to you in the kitchen. Not only can you adapt a recipe from a favorite recipe book, you can experiment and re-create favorite flavors that you love. You can also allow the ingredients to invite you to create a dish. Seeing cucumbers when it begins to get hot out suggests gazpacho to me. Blackberries at the height of summer invite me to create the ultimate decadence, the blackberry cobbler.

Comfort foods speak to you when you are feeling depressed or down. When your life is saying "scarcity" in one way or another, comfort foods reassure you of abundance. A scone recipe, chai, spinach soup, mashed potatoes, tempeh salad, a peanut soup, and a baked tofu—these are my comfort foods and I have included them here. I also gravitate to sauces—mixing something smooth with something chewy speaks to me of abundance.

At the end of the recipes you will find a description of some of the more esoteric ingredients.

Approach vegetarian cooking as an opportunity to experience freedom and joy, rather than as a burden. In *The Inner Art of Vegetarianism,* I offer these suggestions for experiencing the meditative qualities of cooking:

1. When you are cooking, don't listen to the news on radio or TV. The news you are waiting for is coming from within. Cooking is complete within itself.

2. Don't answer the phone. It will interrupt the flow.

3. If there are children around, welcome them into the process.

4. Whether a beginning or experienced vegetarian, write in your recipe books. Interact with the recipes. Date them and write if they worked or you changed anything. Write what you or others thought about them. Writing about the recipe invites you back to it. It reminds you where you've been. You don't have to retrace your steps.

5. If the recipe was great, copy it. Create a "keepers" notebook. Put all your favorite and successful recipes here. This reduces the planning time when you cook them again. You can consult your "keepers" notebook.

6. Plan your meals when you're relaxed and refreshed. If you know your evening energy is rushed, unthinking, and tired, don't leave it until the evening to decide what supper will be. Instead, select the recipe earlier in the day, or before you go to bed the night before. Then, when the time comes, you can step into the process you began earlier.

    or

7. Go shopping and see what vegetables speak to you. Allow the food to express itself in your cooking.

Believe me, if I can progress from having to learn how to handle a pepper to having my meat-eating relatives enjoy my vegan meals, anyone can master these recipes!

Allow the process of vegetarian cooking to transform you. The abundance of vegetarianism can unfold in your own kitchen: abundance of materials in the fresh herbs that you may use in a pasta recipe, abundance in taste in a simple recipe that offers flavors that you relish, abundance in spirit in welcoming others to your vegetarian eating style. The vegetables, fruits, herbs, grains, beans, sea vegetables—all the possible foods and the endless kaleidoscopic possibilities of combinations—will welcome you with abundant possibilities. Enjoy the process!

APPETIZERS AND BEVERAGES

A QUICK DIP

Makes 6 servings as a snack

Mix salsa, chopped cilantro, and Tofutti Better Than Sour Cream Sour Supreme®. Serve with tortilla chips.

PITA CRISPS

Makes 4 servings

These can be used to dip into appetizers or to accompany soups or salads.

    2 pita breads (6 inches in diameter)
    2 teaspoons vegan margarine
    2 teaspoons dried oregano
    4–6 tablespoons nutritional yeast flakes
    6 cloves garlic, diced
    olive oil

1. Preheat the broiler, with the broiler rack about 4 to 5 inches beneath the heating element.
2. Split the pita breads horizontally into two rounds. Place each half, rough side up, onto an ungreased baking sheet. Spread lightly with the margarine.

3. Toss together the oregano, nutritional yeast flakes, and garlic. Sprinkle this mixture over the margarine. Then dribble a little olive oil over it.

4. Broil for about 2 minutes or until the edges are lightly browned. You need to watch them closely so that they do not burn. As they cool, they will get more crispy.

5. Remove from the oven. Use a pizza cutter to cut them into quarters or sixths. And serve.

TOFU PÂTÉ

Makes about 3 cups. Enough for an appetizer at a party or as a spread for sandwiches for 6, or as a comfort food for you for several days.

This is scrumptious. I have adapted it slightly from Joanne Stepaniak's excellent *The Vegan Sourcebook.* First, I doubled the recipe because everyone loves it. I also think it often needs to be thinned slightly so that it looks and feels smooth and luxurious. You can serve it with pita crisps or warmed pita bread.

1 pound firm regular tofu

1 cup shredded carrot

$1/2$ cup sliced scallions

4 tablespoons tahini

2 tablespoons white miso (Joanne uses sweet white miso, I have used mellow white miso).

4 teaspoons tamari

If necessary, a little plain soy milk to thin pâté

1. Steam or simmer the tofu in water for ten minutes. Let cool.
2. While the tofu simmers, prepare the carrots and scallions. Run the carrots through the food processor's grater or grate by hand and set aside.
3. Fit the food processor with a metal blade. Crumble the cooled tofu into it. Add the tahini, miso, and tamari and process into a thick smooth paste. Add a tablespoon or two of soy milk if necessary for smoothness.
4. Add the grated carrot and scallions and briefly pulse until they are evenly distributed. Allow to chill in a container several hours before serving.

ARTICHOKE PUFFS

*Serves 12 as an appetizer. As part of a dinner's
main course, serve two per person.*

These are a variation on an appetizer I first encountered when PETA asked me to endorse one of their early cookbooks, *The Compassionate Cook*. I felt the puffs needed more variety and added mushrooms and pimentos to the artichokes.

Two 10-ounce packages puff pastry shells (12 shells)

1 teaspoon vegan margarine

2 teaspoons water

1/4 cup scallions or finely chopped onions

2 teaspoons cornstarch

1 1/4 cups plain soy milk

8 ounces mushrooms

1 garlic clove, diced

1 tablespoon olive oil

One 14-ounce can artichoke hearts

1 roasted bell pepper, diced (If you don't have a roasted bell pepper on hand, you can use 1/4 cup pimentos from a jar.)

Paprika

Salt and pepper

1. Bake the pastry shells according to the directions on the package.
2. While the shells are baking, heat the margarine and water in a frying pan over medium heat. Add the scallions or onions and cook for 10 minutes, or until they are transparent.
3. Stir in the cornstarch and continue cooking for a few minutes.
4. Add the soy milk and stir until mixture is thickened. Remove from the heat and set aside.
5. Slice the mushrooms and sauté them with the garlic in the olive oil.
6. Drain the artichoke hearts and chop them into bite-size pieces.
7. Add the mushrooms, artichoke hearts, and red pepper or pimentos to the thickened soy milk mixture.
8. Season with paprika, salt, and pepper.
9. Remove the tops from the pastry shells. Set the tops aside. Spoon the creamed mixture into each pastry shell and return them to the oven for 5 minutes at 350 degrees.
10. Replace the tops and serve.

CHAI (SPICED CAFFEINE-FREE TEA)

Yield: About 8 cups

With all the chai on the market, why bother to make your own? Well, first of all, why not? It's fun. I love the smell of cardamom. Many chais contain honey, and almost all of them have caffeine in them. For a caffeine-free, scrumptious drink, try the following. This is a double recipe. Refrigerated, it keeps for about a week, which is how long it takes me to drink it and share it with my friends.

8 cups water

Two 3-inch cinnamon sticks

2-inch piece fresh ginger, cut into 8 slices

1 teaspoon cardamom seeds

1 teaspoon black peppercorns

1 teaspoon whole cloves

2 teaspoons whole coriander seeds

1 teaspoon ground nutmeg

1 quart soy milk

FruitSource or other sweetener to taste

1. Bring the water and spices to boil in a saucepan. Reduce the heat, cover, and simmer for 20 minutes, until the water has reduced by about 50 percent.
2. Add the soy milk and, without bringing to a boil, simmer for 3 or 4 minutes. Turn off the heat and let the spices infuse the soy milk as long as you wish. The longer it sits, the stronger the taste. Pour the chai through a strainer to catch any floating spices. Sweeten to taste and enjoy! Refrigerate the remaining chai and drink warm or cold whenever you wish.

ORANGE JULIUS

This yields six cups, but it is so scrumptious that people often want seconds, thus it may not serve 6.

Here is a way to introduce people to soy milk. Smooth, tasty, and silky.

One 16-ounce can of frozen orange juice (don't defrost)
32 ounces vanilla soy milk
Sweetener (optional)
1 tablespoon vanilla
ice cubes

1. Empty the frozen orange juice into a blender.
2. Fill the orange juice container twice with soy milk. I add a couple of tablespoons of Sucanat™, too.
3. Blend together. Let it get thoroughly mixed and frothy.
4. Add the vanilla, a few ice cubes, and pulverize.

BREAKFASTS AND QUICK LUNCHES

GRANOLA

Yield: Approximately 8 cups granola

Don't let the number of ingredients daunt you. While this makes a wonderful granola, you can leave out many of the ingredients and have quite a satisfactory breakfast. Just don't omit the oats, the sweetener, or the oil. Everything else is negotiable to your taste buds.

This granola can be eaten as a snack, packed in containers for traveling, and, of course, served for breakfast with soy milk and fresh fruit. My favorite is pineapple.

4 cups old-fashioned rolled oats (not quick-cooking oats)

$^3/_4$ cup raw pumpkin seeds

$^3/_4$ cup unsalted raw sunflower seeds

$^1/_4$ cup sesame seeds

1 cup coarsely chopped unblanched almonds

1 cup coarsely chopped unblanched walnuts

$^1/_2$ cup wheat germ

$^1/_4$ cup wheat bran

$^1/_2$ cup powdered soy milk (I use powdered Better Than
    Milk® Soy Light Beverage Mix from Fuller Life, Inc.)

1 tablespoon ground cinnamon

2 teaspoons ground nutmeg

$^1/_4$ teaspoon ground cloves

Zest of 1 orange, finely grated

$^1/_2$ cup safflower oil

$^1/_2$ cup maple syrup

$^1/_2$ cup barley malt syrup

1 tablespoon vanilla extract

1 to 2 teaspoons almond extract

1. Preheat the oven to 350 degrees.

2. In a large mixing bowl, stir together the oats, seeds, almonds, walnuts, wheat germ, wheat bran, powdered soy milk, cinnamon, nutmeg, cloves, and orange zest.

3. In a small saucepan over medium heat, stir together the oil, maple syrup, and barley malt syrup. Remove from the heat and stir in the vanilla and almond extracts.

4. Pour the contents of the saucepan over the oat mixture and toss with your hands until all the ingredients are evenly moistened. (Use a wooden spoon if you prefer, but your hands do the job better and there is something very satisfying about the mixing process.)

5. Spread on 2 cookie sheets, press evenly, and bake for 30 minutes, stirring every ten minutes. Be sure to loosen the edges and mix them into the middle; otherwise the edges will brown too quickly. At 20 minutes, check every 3–4 minutes. Remove once the mixture is *light* brown.

6. Remove from the oven, and let cool in the pan.

7. When the granola has cooled to room temperature, break it into chunks and then smaller pieces. At this point you can add 2 cups of dried fruit of your choice (cherries, blueberries, raisins, figs, apricots). Some prefer not to add the dried fruit until they are actually eating the granola because they feel its moistness dampens the granola as it is sitting in the bags or tins or other containers into which you will put the baked and cooled granola.

SOURDOUGH PANCAKES AND WAFFLES

Serves 4

While these pancakes take some advance planning, they are very quick to prepare. Because they rise so magnificently and so quickly, they are fun to prepare and quickly convert people to this simple vegan recipe. I adapted this from the marvelous Jennifer Raymond, whose *The Peaceful Palate* first introduced me to this use of sourdough. If you don't have a sourdough culture, you can buy a powdered mix at health food stores and follow the directions for activating it. This is your "starter." Then keep it refrigerated until you need it. The directions for awakening the culture are adapted from Ed Wood's *World Sourdoughs from Antiquity*.

Awakening the Starter

Sourdough starter

4 cups white flour

water

1. Twenty-four hours before you wish to serve the pancakes, take your sourdough starter out of the refrigerator. Place it in a large bowl. Feed it 1 cup of flour and ¾ cup of warm water (75–85 degrees). You do not have to make this mixture lump-free. Warm the culture by keeping it at about 80–85 degrees. (On top of your water heater is one place for anyone with an electric stove. Otherwise, above a gas stove's pilot light is fine.) Leave for 6 to 8 hours or overnight. The starter should now be bubbling.

2. Once your starter has awakened, add 2 cups of warm water and mix briefly. Then add 3 cups flour, a cup at a time, mixing briefly between cups. Cover the bowl with plastic wrap and then a dry cloth. Leave for about 12 hours. It is possible to do this step in a shorter amount of time. Shorter fermentations produce a milder flavor. Remember to reserve at least one cup of sourdough as your next starter.

For the Pancakes or Waffles

3 cups sourdough starter

$1\frac{1}{2}$ teaspoons baking soda

$2\frac{1}{2}$ tablespoons sweetener (I use Sucanat™)

$1\frac{1}{2}$ tablespoons oil (not olive)

$\frac{1}{3}$ cup wheat germ

Freshly ground cinnamon, if possible, or $\frac{1}{2}$ teaspoon
  powdered cinnamon

1. Put the sourdough culture in a large mixing bowl. In a small bowl, mix together the baking soda, sweetener, wheat germ, oil, and cinnamon. Stir this into the sourdough mixture. If you have young kids, invite them to do this. They will be thrilled by the reaction of the sourdough to the baking soda.
2. Drop the pancake mix onto a hot, lightly greased griddle or pan. I use an ice cream scoop.
3. Cook until the pancakes are light brown and puffed up. Flip over and cook the other side. Serve immediately.

For waffles: Follow the instructions for your waffle maker. The batter is perfect for waffles and makes light, beautiful, perfect waffles every time.

Burgers

Select your favorite frozen veggie burger. Prepare and serve with lettuce, sprouts, tomatoes, broiled portobello mushrooms, vegetarian Yves Canadian "bacon," dill pickles. For variation, serve on bagels rather than buns.

Falafel

A box of Fantastic Falafel yields servings for 8

Falafel mix or frozen falafel
Oil for frying

1. Follow instructions for reconstituting falafel or for baking frozen falafels.
2. Form small patties using 3–4 tablespoons of falafel if using a mix.
3. Over medium heat, in just enough oil to keep them from sticking, sauté patties until golden and crispy. Turn once.

Tahini Sauce

$\frac{1}{2}$ **cup tahini**
$\frac{1}{4}$ **cup lemon juice**
$\frac{1}{2}$ **cup water**

Mix ingredients together.
Serve falafel in pita bread with diced tomatoes, shredded lettuce, cucumber, and dill pickles, if desired. Then drizzle tahini sauce into the stuffed pita.

TEMPEH SALAD SANDWICH

Makes 4 sandwiches

I like preparing the tempeh salad in advance the night before. This is one of my favorite comfort foods. I usually make a double recipe to save time.

> 8 ounces tempeh
> ¼ cup Follow Your Heart Vegenaise® (Vegenaise® is the
>   best vegan mayonnaise!)
> 2 tablespoons nutritional yeast flakes
> 3 tablespoons chopped dill pickle
> 2 tablespoons minced parsley
> 1 teaspoon mustard
> 1 teaspoon tamari
> 1 stalk celery
> ¼ medium onion, chopped, or ¼ cup diced scallions

1. Break the tempeh in half and steam in a vegetable steamer for 20 minutes. Let it cool. Crumble it into a bowl.
2. Combine remaining ingredients and mix them into the crumbled tempeh. Cover and chill. Serve in pita bread with butter lettuce and tomatoes.

MAIN DISHES

PASTA WITH PEANUT SAUCE

Makes 8 servings

This is a perennial favorite and variations of it can be found in countless vegetarian cookbooks. You can use somen noodles or your choice of spaghetti noodles. You can have it as a cold salad or hot. This peanut sauce differs from the one in the sauces section, and I include both because each has its strengths.

Peanut Sauce

6 cloves garlic

1 bunch cilantro, leaves and upper stems

1 inch fresh ginger, peeled

1 tablespoon peanut oil

1 tablespoon sesame oil

1 tablespoon hot chili oil

$\frac{1}{2}$ cup peanut butter

$\frac{1}{2}$ cup soy sauce

3 tablespoons Sucanat or other sweetener

3 tablespoons rice wine vinegar

Put the garlic, cilantro, and ginger in food processor with metal blade and process until finely chopped. Add the oils, peanut butter, soy sauce, and sweetener. Process to combine all the ingredients, stopping and scraping down the sides a couple of times. Add the vinegar to taste. Adjust seasonings if necessary. You can thin the sauce with hot water if it is too thick.

Noodles

1 pound noodles

2 tablespoons sesame oil

$\frac{1}{2}$ cup chopped cilantro leaves

6 scallions

1 recipe Golden Fried Tofu (page 253)

1. Cook your noodles until al dente. If you are having cold noodles, pour them into a colander once they are done and rinse them with cold water. Shake the excess water off and place in a large bowl.

2. Toss with the sesame oil, cilantro, and scallions. Just before serving, add the peanut sauce and the tofu.

MUSHROOM COBBLER

Serves 8

As I said at the beginning of this chapter, mushrooms and cobblers both convey a sense of abundance to me. Combining them results in a delicious and impressive main course. It is always received with enthusiasm when I prepare it for celebrations or holidays. This is an adaptation of a recipe from Anna Thomas's *The New Vegetarian Epicure*. While Thomas emphasizes more exotic mushrooms, this cobbler is fine if you use portobello and cremini mushrooms. Be aware: this is a time-consuming recipe, as there are three steps: creating the filling, making the sauce, and making the topping.

Filling

1 pound red Spanish onions (Thomas calls for 2 pounds,
    and some may feel that 1 pound is still too much.
    Modify accordingly.)
$2^{1}/_{2}$ tablespoons olive oil
$2^{1}/_{2}$ tablespoons vegan margarine
Salt to taste
1 ounce dried porcini mushrooms
about $^{1}/_{3}$ to $^{1}/_{2}$ cup boiling water
$^{1}/_{2}$ pound fresh porcini or portobello mushrooms
$^{1}/_{2}$ pound fresh oyster mushrooms or cremini mushrooms

Sauce

2 cloves garlic, chopped

Pinch dried thyme

Pinch cayenne

Freshly ground black pepper

$\frac{1}{2}$ cup dry red wine (nonalcoholic wine works just fine)

$1\frac{1}{2}$ tablespoons flour

$1\frac{1}{2}$ cups plain soy milk, heated

Cobbler

$1\frac{1}{3}$ cup plain soy milk

1 tablespoon cider vinegar

1 cup white flour

1 cup pastry flour or spelt flour

1 teaspoon baking soda

$1\frac{1}{2}$ teaspoon baking powder

1 teaspoon salt

4 tablespoons Spectrum Spread (other brands don't seem to work as well)

4 tablespoons nutritional yeast flakes, lightly toasted over low heat

Prepare the Filling and Sauce

1. Peel, quarter, and slice the red onions.
2. In a large nonstick pan, heat a tablespoon of olive oil and a tablespoon of the soy margarine. Add the onions and some salt, and cook over low heat.

3. Let the onions cook for about an hour, stirring them often as you prepare the other ingredients. The onions will soften and then caramelize:
   they will turn golden-brown and should become intensely sweet.

4. Pour the boiling water over the dried porcini and let them soak for at
   least 30 minutes.

5. Clean, trim, and slice the fresh mushrooms.

6. When the dried porcini are soft, remove them from the water and
   reserve the water. Rinse the mushrooms and chop them finely. Strain
   the water through a coffee filter or cheesecloth and put aside.

7. In another large nonstick skillet, heat $1\frac{1}{2}$ tablespoons of olive oil and
   $\frac{1}{2}$ tablespoons vegan margarine.

8. Add the chopped garlic and stir for 1 minute so that the garlic can begin
   to release its flavor. Add the sliced fresh mushrooms and a little salt.

9. Sauté the mushrooms over medium heat, stirring frequently.

10. When they begin to release their liquid, add the porcini, thyme,
    cayenne, and black pepper, and cook over medium heat until the liq-
    uid the mushrooms released has cooked away and the mushrooms are
    sizzling.

11. Add the red wine, stirring as it cooks away, and then add the soaking
    liquid from the dried mushrooms. Once you have stirred this in, and
    the mushrooms are a thick, bubbling mass, combine them with the
    caramelized onions. Simmer them together for a few minutes.

12. As the onions caramelize, slowly heat the soy milk for the sauce.

13. Melt the remaining tablespoon of soy margarine in a small saucepan.
    Stir in $1\frac{1}{2}$ tablespoons flour. Stir together for 3 or 4 minutes, until
    mixture is golden.

14. Slowly add the heated milk, whisking the mixture as you do so. Keep
    stirring with a whisk as the sauce thickens. This may take several min-
    utes. Once the mushroom-onion mixture has simmered for a few
    minutes, add the sauce to it.

15. Taste, and adjust the seasonings. I usually find that this mixture needs a little more salt, pepper, and cayenne (but just a pinch more of the latter). You can refrigerate this mixture overnight.

16. When ready to bake the mushroom cobbler, pour the mushroom mixture into a lightly oiled gratin dish or a rectangular baking dish, spreading it evenly.

Prepare the Cobbler Dough

1. Preheat the oven to 400 degrees.

2. Put the cider vinegar into a measuring cup that can hold at least $1\frac{1}{3}$ cups of liquid. Pour the soy milk into the measuring cup until it measures $1\frac{1}{3}$ cups. Let this sit as you work with the dry ingredients. The vinegar acts on the soy milk so that it becomes like buttermilk.

3. Combine the flours, baking soda, baking powder, and salt in a medium-size bowl. Using a pastry cutter or a fork, add the Spectrum Spread until the mixture is like coarse cornmeal. Add the nutritional yeast flakes.

4. Quickly stir in the soy milk. Don't overmix it. As soon as a thick and sticky dough forms, spoon it onto the mushroom mixture. Bake the cobbler for about 25 minutes. The topping should be lightly golden brown and a toothpick when inserted into it should come out clean.

    Serve hot, with a green salad.

NEAT LOAF

Serves 8 to 10

From the ingenious Jennifer Raymond's *The Peaceful Palate.* This is a continual hands-down meat eaters' favorite. Sliced leftovers make great sandwiches. Jennifer recommends using a food processor for this recipe. She is right. It quickly makes each ingredient the right size for mixing together.

> 1 cup cooked brown rice
>
> 1 cup wheat germ
>
> 1 cup quick rolled oats or oat bran (Whiz oats in a dry
>   food processor for your own oat bran)
>
> 1 cup finely chopped walnuts or sunflower seeds
>
> 1 cup chopped mushrooms
>
> 1 onion, finely chopped
>
> $1/2$ medium bell pepper, finely chopped
>
> 1 medium carrot, shredded or finely chopped
>
> $1/2$ teaspoon each: thyme, marjoram, sage
>
> 2 tablespoons soy sauce
>
> 2 tablespoons stone-ground or Dijon-style mustard
>
> 1 tablespoon peanut butter

Note: Some adapt this recipe by adding a little tomato paste to the mix. Jennifer puts ketchup on the top for the last twenty minutes, but this variation was soundly rejected by my tasters.

1. Preheat the oven to 350 degrees.
2. Combine all ingredients and mix for 2 minutes with a large spoon to help to bind together.
3. Pat into a greased 5 × 9–inch loaf pan, and bake for an hour, or until lightly browned. Let stand 10 minutes before serving.

BAKED WALNUT BALLS BÉCHAMEL

Yield: About 20–25 walnut balls

The caterer hired in 1978 to cater our wedding reception borrowed some of my vegetarian cookbooks in his search for mouthwatering main courses for the event. He discovered Baked Walnut and Cheddar Balls Béchamel in Anna Thomas's *The Vegetarian Epicure*. The day of the wedding he told me that it was this recipe that convinced him to get a food processor. (It was 1978, after all!) The walnut balls looked gorgeous swimming in the sauce in a chafing dish. At the reception, one of the die-hard, I'm-a-meat-eater-and-proud-of-it guests dished some walnut balls onto his plate and shouted to me, "I'm glad you are serving meat here!" Little did he know!

When I became a vegan, I dropped these favorites from my recipe file. But Mary Hunt shared a well-used copy of Reggi Norton and Martha Wagner's *The Soy of Cooking,* and the Walnut Balls with Tofu Lemon Cream Sauce reminded me of Anna Thomas's delectable treats.

The following variation combines the best from each of these books: Thomas uses onions; Norton and Wagner scallions. Silken tofu easily replaces the eggs of the original. But I think a béchamel sauce is smoother and I have veganized Thomas's original rather than follow the example of a tofu cream sauce.

For the walnut balls

1½ cups toasted ground walnuts
¼ cup bread crumbs
½ cup wheat germ
3 tablespoons chopped parsley
½ cup minced onion
6 ounces silken tofu
¼ cup plus 1 tablespoon soy milk
¼ cup whole wheat flour
3 cloves garlic
¼ cup toasted nutritional yeast flakes
½ teaspoon prepared mustard
½ teaspoon salt
1 teaspoon lemon juice
Freshly ground pepper to taste

1. In a large bowl, combine the ground walnuts, bread crumbs, wheat germ, parsley, and minced onion.
2. Combine the remaining ingredients in a food processor until smooth. Mix into the walnut mixture.
3. The mixture should be moist but able to hold its shape. Roll the mixture into walnut-size balls, and place on an oiled baking sheet.
4. Bake at 350 degrees for about 30 to 40 minutes. The bottoms of the balls should be lightly browned.

Make the béchamel sauce while the walnut balls bake.

243

Béchamel Sauce

3 tablespoons canola or other light unflavored oil

1/2 cup minced onion

3 tablespoons whole wheat pastry flour

3 cups hot (but not boiling) plain soy milk

1 teaspoon peppercorns

1/2 teaspoon thyme

1 small bay leaf

Pinch nutmeg (freshly grated if possible)

Salt to taste

Dash cayenne

1. Heat the oil over medium heat until hot. Turn the heat to medium-low, add the onion, and sauté for 3 to 4 minutes. Add the flour and stir it in. It will immediately clump up. Allow the mixture to cook for a few minutes while stirring it.

2. Add the soy milk slowly into the flour mixture, stirring with a whisk as you do. At first it will thicken as soon as the liquid is added; watch for lumps and beat them out with your whisk. Slowly, as more liquid is added, it will thin out, but it will thicken again over the next few minutes.

3. When all of the liquid has been stirred in, add peppercorns, thyme, the bay leaf, nutmeg, and salt. Let the sauce cook slowly for 10 to 15 minutes, stirring once in a while. Pour it into its serving bowl using a sieve, to eliminate the surprise of peppercorns and bay leaf. If you don't want to be bothered with a sieve, retrieve those elusive peppercorns and the bay leaf with a spoon. The sauce should be thickened, creamy, and tasty. Add a dash of cayenne at the end.

Remove the walnut balls from the oven, place in a serving dish, and pour the béchamel sauce over them. Serve piping hot!

ROASTED VEGETABLES WITH GARLIC AND FENNEL SEEDS

Serves 8–10

Adapted from Ken Bergeron's *Professional Vegetarian Cooking.* At the 2000 World Vegetarian Congress, Ken Bergeron and I were both waiting for an elevator. There was just enough time for me to exude about this recipe and how I use it with tofu for an evening meal. He was gracious and generous in encouraging me to include it in this book. This recipe—and its originator—both reveal abundance. You will enjoy variations of this recipe throughout the cold winter months.

> ¼ cup olive oil
>
> 1 tablespoon crushed garlic
>
> 1 tablespoon fennel seeds
>
> ½ teaspoon salt
>
> Pinch ground black pepper
>
> 1½ pounds butternut squash, peeled and cut into 1-inch chunks
>
> 1½ pounds carrots, cut into 1-inch chunks
>
> 1 pound small red onions, quartered
>
> 1½ pounds parsnips
>
> 3 tablespoons chopped fresh parsley
>
> 1 tablespoon balsamic vinegar
>
> 1 pound Tasty Tofu, cubed (see page 256).

1. Preheat oven to 425 degrees.
2. Mix 1 tablespoon of the olive oil with the garlic and fennel seeds and set aside.

3. Toss vegetables with the remaining olive oil and salt and pepper. Place vegetables on a large baking sheet, with the harder vegetables around the outside, surrounding the softer vegetables. Bake for 15 minutes.

4. Stir and loosen vegetables if they have begun to stick to the pan. Roast 15 minutes longer or until they are tender when a fork pierces them.

5. Toss vegetables with the olive oil, garlic, and fennel seeds. Roast for 8 minutes. Toss vegetables with the chopped parsley and balsamic vinegar. Bake for 2 more minutes. Remove from the oven.

6. Toss with the Tasty Tofu and serve.

STUFF-YOUR-OWN TORTILLAS

My children love this meal.

Gather a variety of ingredients and let each person make their own tortillas. Here are some of our favorites.

Sautéed mushrooms
Tasty Tofu (see page 256)
Roasted red pepper
Fresh tomatoes
Lettuce
Tofutti Better Than Sour Cream
Salsa
Sun-dried tomatoes

(CHICKEN-APPROVED)
CHICKENLESS NUGGETS

About 50 nuggets

Adapted from Karen Davis, president of United Poultry Concerns, P.O. Box 150, Machipongo, Virginia, 23405, www.upc-online.org

1 box White Wave Chicken Style Wheat Meat
$\frac{1}{2}$ cup flour
$\frac{1}{2}$ cup bread crumbs
2 cloves garlic, minced
Salt and pepper to taste
1 teaspoon oregano
1 teaspoon parsley
$\frac{1}{2}$ teaspoon thyme
$\frac{1}{2}$ teaspoon basil
$\frac{1}{2}$ teaspoon paprika
Soy milk for dipping
Olive (or other vegetable) oil for frying
Favorite bottled or homemade spaghetti sauce

1. Preheat oven to 375 degrees.
2. Defrost Wheat Meat and cut into bite-size nuggets.
3. Mix flour and bread crumbs with salt, pepper, garlic, and Italian seasonings.
4. Dip Wheat Meat nuggets into soy milk and then into bread crumb mixture. This mixture gets increasingly bound together as you work with it. I have tried two alternatives: a) dip the nuggets into a part of this mixture, and keep the rest dry until needed, or b) separate the flour from the bread crumb mix, and dip the nuggets into the flour, then the soy milk, then the bread crumb mix.

5. Fry nuggets in oil until golden brown.

6. Cover the bottom of a baking dish with a layer of spaghetti sauce. Place nuggets on top. Pour another layer of sauce over nuggets.

7. Bake for 20–30 minutes.

Turnovers

Yield: 6 turnovers

1 box Wheat Meat (chicken style)

1 tablespoon vegan margarine

Salt and pepper to taste

$1/2$ package puff pastry sheets (1 sheet) ($17^1/_2$-ounce size)

$1^1/_2$ teaspoons Ener-G Egg Replacer or cornstarch

2 tablespoons water

Flour for working surface

1 container Tofutti Better Than Cream Cheese, herb flavor
(If you can only get plain, add 2 tablespoons fresh basil to the chopped parsley.)

$1/2$ cup chopped parsley

1. Defrost Wheat Meat and cut into bite-size nuggets. Fry lightly in the margarine. Season with a little salt and pepper. Let cool.

2. Thaw pastry sheet at room temperature for 30 minutes. Mix Egg Replacer or cornstarch with the water. Preheat oven to 400 degrees.

3. Unfold pastry on lightly floured surface. Roll out until it is a 14-inch square and cut into 6 squares. Spread about 2 tablespoons of Better Than Cream Cheese in the center of each square. Sprinkle with about 1 tablespoon parsley and top with the cooled Wheat Meat. Brush edges of squares with water mixture. Fold each corner to the center and seal edges. Place seam side down on baking sheet. Brush again with the water mixture.

4. Bake 25 minutes or until golden.

SHEPHERD'S PIE

Serves 8

This pie is heartily recommended for those who cook for meat eaters.

- 1 cup dried lentils (green or brown), or 2 cups cooked lentils
- 1 large yellow onion, chopped
- 2 carrots, chopped
- ½ cup celery, sliced
- 2 cloves garlic, chopped
- Olive oil for sautéing
- 1 teaspoon mixed dried herbs (marjoram, thyme, basil, sage—your choice)
- One 8-ounce can tomato sauce or one 15-ounce can tomatoes, chopped
- 2 tablespoons soy sauce
- 2–3 tablespoons chopped parsley
- Salt and black pepper
- 4 medium potatoes, cooked and mashed
- Paprika
- 2 tablespoons nutritional yeast flakes

1. If the lentils are uncooked, boil them in water for 45 minutes. Drain.
2. Preheat oven to 350 degrees. Sauté onion, carrots, celery, and garlic in a little olive oil until softened.
3. Add herbs, tomatoes, soy sauce, lentils, parsley, and salt and pepper to taste. Stir.
4. Spoon mixture into a lightly oiled baking dish. Spread mashed potatoes evenly over the top, drawing a fork over the surface to make ridges. Sprinkle paprika and nutritional yeast flakes on top of potatoes.
5. Bake 45 minutes, until golden brown.

FAVORITE TOFU RECIPES

BAKED TOFU

Yield: 6 baked slices

From Mary Lou Randour, author of *Animal Grace*.

You can vary the seasonings by adding pepper flakes or making your own bread crumbs.

1 pound regular tofu
1 cup of Italian bread crumbs. Or make your own and
  flavor them to your liking.
1 tablespoon nutritional yeast flakes
$\frac{1}{3}$ cup soy milk or tamari

1. Remove the tofu from the water and wrap it in something absorbent. Press it between two plates for 24 hours.
2. Preheat oven to 350 degrees.
3. Stand tofu on its side and cut it into three slices. Then cut it diagonally.
4. Mix the bread crumbs with the nutritional yeast flakes.
5. Dip the tofu triangles into the soy milk or tamari. Then dip them into the bread crumbs.
6. Bake for twenty minutes, turning the tofu once. Experiment with the baking time if you want it crisper.

TOFU STEAKS

*Yield: 8 slices. Or, once cooked, cut into cubes and
add to pasta.*

Delicious with pasta dishes.

1 pound firm regular tofu
2 tablespoons soy sauce
2 tablespoons wine vinegar
1½ tablespoons oil

1. Slice tofu into 8 slices.
2. Marinate the tofu slices in the soy sauce, vinegar, and 1 tablespoon oil for several hours.
3. Heat a nonstick skillet, and add ½ tablespoon oil. Cook 4 slices in the oil and half of the marinade. When both sides are browned, remove from the skillet and cook the other 4 slices in the remaining marinade. If all of the marinade is absorbed during cooking, add a little more vinegar and olive oil to the pan.

GOLDEN FRIED TOFU

Serves 3–4

1 pound firm regular tofu
2 tablespoons peanut oil

1. Drain the tofu and wrap it in a clean kitchen towel. Let it sit for ten to thirty minutes.
2. Remove tofu from the towel and cut into six slices. Cut each slice diagonally in half. You will now have twelve triangles. If you have a skillet that can hold all the triangles, heat the oil and then add the tofu. Otherwise, heat 1 tablespoon of the oil in a skillet (preferably nonstick) over medium-high heat. Add the tofu triangles and fry them for several minutes, until they are golden in color. They should not get dried out or hardened. Turn the triangles over and fry the other side. Remove to a plate covered with two paper towels. Add the remaining 1 tablespoon oil and cook the remaining tofu triangles.

CRISPED CREAMY TOFU

Serves 4

Adapted by my friend Amie Hamlin, director and founder of Club Veg, a vegetarian education and travel group. The original recipe appeared in *Veggie Life* magazine, March 1994, featuring recipes from It's Only Natural Restaurant in Lititz, Pennsylvania. A meat-eating friend of mine could not get enough of this easy-to-prepare dish!

> ¼ cup light miso (Mellow White or chickpea)
> 2 tablespoons frozen orange juice concentrate
> 1 tablespoon sesame seeds
> 1 pound firm or extra-firm regular tofu, drained

1. Preheat the oven to 475 degrees.
2. As the piece of tofu sits on your cutting board, quarter it in slices parallel to the counter, so that you have 4 pieces that are the size of the largest surface of the tofu. Slice the tofu diagonally to make 8 triangles.
3. In a small bowl, combine miso and orange juice concentrate.
4. Lightly roast sesame seeds in a dry skillet until nutty smelling and golden brown, about 3 minutes.
5. Place tofu on a lightly oiled baking sheet and spread with the miso topping. Sprinkle each piece with sesame seeds.
6. Bake for 8 to 10 minutes, until golden brown.

TOFU CUBES

Serves 2 to 3

Mmm! Delicious! Add to salads or pastas or tortillas or eat right from the frying pan.

- 1 pound firm regular tofu
- 3 tablespoons nutritional yeast flakes
- 2 tablespoons flour
- 1 teaspoon garlic powder
- 1 teaspoon pepper
- $\frac{1}{2}$ teaspoon paprika
- 1 teaspoon powdered vegetarian stock
- 1–2 tablespoons oil

1. Cut tofu into cubes about $\frac{1}{4}$ inch. Do not pat them dry.
2. Combine all the other ingredients except the oil in a container with a lid. Add the tofu, put the lid on, and shake well to coat the tofu.
3. Heat oil in a nonstick skillet. Add the tofu and cook over medium heat, turning the tofu every few minutes until it is golden brown and crispy.

Tasty Tofu

Yield: 12 slices

A versatile way to prepare tofu—use it with roasted vegetables, sauté it with veggies, stick into stews.

> 2 pounds firm regular tofu
> 1/3 cup tamari or soy sauce
> 2 tablespoons maple syrup

1. Preheat the oven to 400 degrees. Use parchment paper to line a baking pan.
2. Drain the tofu. Wrap it in a towel for about 15 minutes to absorb excess moisture.
3. Cut the tofu in half, and then in thirds along the width. You will have 12 slices about 1/2 inch thick.
4. In a pie plate, combine the maple syrup and the tamari. Dip the tofu in this mixture and place on the parchment paper. Bake for 20 to 25 minutes, until it is lightly browned.
5. Turn the tofu over with a spatula. It may stick slightly to the parchment paper, but loosen it slowly so that you will not lose the "skin" it develops. Brush the tofu with any of the remaining maple syrup–tamari mixture, and bake for 20 minutes or until it is a luscious brown. Let cool. Use within 3 days; keep stored in an airtight container in the refrigerator.

SOUPS AND HEARTY SAUCES

GAZPACHO

*Serves 6. As a main course, accompanied by a
favorite tofu recipe, serves 4.*

I think of this as "salad in a soup bowl."

1 cucumber, peeled
1 green bell pepper, seeded and quartered
$\frac{1}{2}$ cup water
1 tablespoon "chicken flavor" vegetable powdered stock
One 28-ounce can tomatoes
4–5 tablespoons olive oil
$\frac{1}{2}$ cup parsley
6–8 sprigs basil
3–4 cloves garlic
1 small onion, peeled and quartered
Dash or two of Tabasco or other hot sauce
Salt and pepper to taste
$\frac{1}{4}$ cup red wine vinegar
4 scallions
Handful cherry tomatoes
Croutons

1. Prepare the vegetables. To prepare the cucumber, slice it in half lengthwise, and then slice each half lengthwise in half. Deseed. (A spoon is a
   good tool for this. Run the spoon down the spine of the cucumber.)
   Set aside one-quarter of the green pepper and of the cucumber.
2. Bring the water to a boil, and add the vegetable stock to it. Set aside.

3. Empty the canned tomatoes and their juices into a blender or food processor. Add 4 tablespoons olive oil, parsley, basil, garlic, the stock, hot sauce, salt, pepper, and vinegar. Process until smooth. Empty $3/4$ of the contents of the blender/processor into a pitcher or bowl. Add the onion, the green pepper, and the cucumber (except for the part that you reserved). Pulse briefly, so that the vegetables remain chewy but small. Do not liquefy. It should not be pureed but chunky.

4. Add this to the mixture in the bowl or pitcher. Refrigerate for several hours, so that the flavors meld.

5. Before serving, dice the scallions, the reserved green pepper, and cucumber. Chop the cherry tomatoes in half. Place each of these vegetables in its own small bowl for garnishes (I use Asian teacups), and put the croutons in a larger bowl.

6. Taste the soup and adjust seasonings. It should taste lively. It may need more pepper and salt or another dash of Tabasco. I mix an additional tablespoon of olive oil in at this time.

7. Serve in bowls, letting each guest add the finely minced veggies and croutons to their own soup.

KALE SOUP

4 servings

A fast, delicious way to prepare kale. A cooked, diced potato or squares of toasted bread and minced cilantro leaves are wonderful additions when you serve the soup.

About 3 cups roughly chopped kale leaves

2 tablespoons olive or peanut oil

1 cup minced onion

2 tablespoons minced garlic

One 32-ounce box Imagine No-Chicken Broth

1 tablespoon soy sauce

Salt

1. Strip the leaves from the kale stalk, rinse, and then chop.
2. Place the oil in a large, deep saucepan or soup pot and turn the heat to medium-high. Add the onion and cook until it begins to brown, about 5 to 8 minutes. Stir occasionally.
3. When the onion is golden and tender, add the garlic. Cook 1 minute, then add the broth. Bring to a boil, then lower the heat and add the soy sauce.
4. Add the kale to the simmering broth and cook until it is tender, about 10 minutes. Taste, add salt or soy sauce to adjust seasonings, and serve.

COMFORTING SPINACH SOUP

Serves 3

There is nothing like this soup to say "I care about you" to a visiting friend, and to care for yourself on a day when you need a sense of abundant love. This is adapted from Laurel Robertson's *Laurel's Kitchen Caring*.

3 cups plain soy milk

1 bunch spinach (When cooked, drained, and chopped, it
   will be about $\frac{1}{2}$ cup.)

2 tablespoons vegan margarine

2 tablespoons whole wheat pastry flour

1 small onion

6–10 whole cloves, depending on your taste

$\frac{1}{2}$ to $\frac{3}{4}$ teaspoon salt

Dash nutmeg

1. Warm soy milk in a saucepan.
2. Wash spinach, and leave on the water that clings to it after washing. Put the spinach in a large saucepan over medium-high heat, cook spinach until it wilts, no more than 5 minutes. Drain. (I leave the spinach in the colander to cool as I proceed with making the creamy soup base.)
3. In a separate, heavy pan, melt soy margarine and add flour; heat, stirring a minute or two to cook the flour. Don't let it brown.
4. Add the warm soy milk and stir with attention until the mixture comes almost to a boil and begins to thicken. Don't let it boil.
5. Peel and trim the onion. Stick the cloves into the onion and put the onion into the soy milk sauce. Add salt and nutmeg. Simmer over the lowest possible heat for about a half an hour. Stir every once in a while to make sure the sauce does not stick to the bottom of the pan. Then remove and discard the onion and its cloves.

6. When the spinach has cooled, squeeze out excess liquid and chop the spinach.

7. Blend the spinach in a blender with about 1 cup of the sauce. Then add this to the rest of the sauce. Correct the seasonings; it may need more nutmeg or salt.

Serve with "buttermilk" biscuits (see page 286) and enjoy.

CHEDDARY CHEEZE SOUP

Yield: 5 cups

Meat eaters and vegetarians can't believe this is vegan. It is delicious as a soup or it can be used as a fondue dip for breads and vegetables. Adapted from Joanne Stepaniak's *Vegan Vittles*.

1 medium potato, peeled and quartered
1 large carrot, peeled and coarsely chopped
1 medium onion, peeled and quartered
1 cup water
1 12-ounce package firm silken tofu, crumbled
$1/2$ cup nutritional yeast flakes
2 tablespoons fresh lemon juice
2 tablespoons "chicken flavor" vegetarian stock powder
1 cup plain nondairy milk (I like Vitasoy Creamy Original
   or Unsweetened soymilk)

1. Place the chunks of potato, carrot, and onion in the water in a 2-quart saucepan. Bring to a boil. Reduce heat to medium, cover with a lid, and simmer the vegetables, stirring occasionally, for 10 minutes. They should be tender.

2. Puree the soup. The easiest way to do this is with an immersion (hand) blender. Or, transfer the cooked vegetables, the cooking water, and the remaining ingredients except the milk to a food processor. Process until the mixture is completely smooth.

3. Return the blended soup to the saucepan and stir in the milk. Turn the heat to low and warm the soup, stirring often.

AFRICAN BEAN SOUP

Serves 6

This is from the talented Jennifer Raymond, author of *The Peaceful Palate* and *Fat-Free and Easy*. When she sent this recipe to me, she wrote "Mmm!" next to it. I added "Great!" These exclamations say it all. I serve it with my Golden Fried Tofu.

3 tablespoons soy sauce

1 onion, sliced

2 small sweet potatoes or yams, peeled and diced (about
   2 cups)

1 large carrot, thinly sliced

1 celery stalk, thinly sliced

1 red or green bell pepper, diced

One 15-ounce can crushed tomatoes

3–4 cups vegetable stock (I use Imagine No-Chicken
   Broth)

One 15-ounce can garbanzo beans

$\frac{1}{2}$ cup chopped fresh cilantro

$\frac{1}{3}$–$\frac{1}{2}$ cup peanut butter (I use $\frac{1}{2}$ cup)

1–2 teaspoons curry powder

1 tablespoon tamari or soy sauce

1 recipe Golden Fried Tofu (page 253)

1. Heat $\frac{1}{2}$ cup water and the soy sauce in a large pot. Add onion and sweet potatoes. Cook over medium-high heat, stirring occasionally, for 5 minutes.

2. Stir in carrot, celery, and bell pepper. Check the water. If the pan is almost dry, add a little more water. Cover and continue cooking another 3 minutes, stirring occasionally.

3. Add the tomatoes, stock, garbanzo beans, and cilantro.

4. Blend the peanut butter with $\frac{1}{3}$ cup water and add to the soup along with the curry powder. Stir to mix. Bring to a simmer, then cover and cook ten minutes. Add tamari.

Serve with Golden Fried Tofu and brown rice.

ASIAN NOODLE SOUP

Serves 6

This can be a main-course meal. My family likes it served with some rice.

   1 large piece kombu, about 4 inches by 6 inches

   ⅓ cup soy sauce

   5 teaspoons mirin

   4 teaspoons Sucanat or other sweetener

   12 small or 6–8 large dried shiitake mushrooms

   1 tablespoon canola or peanut oil

   2 tablespoons minced garlic

   4 ounces udon noodles

   2 tablespoons minced ginger

   1 recipe Golden Fried Tofu (page 253)

   4 scallions, minced

   Any of the following: asparagus tips, fresh tomatoes, two
      handfuls of fresh spinach, snow peas, or your favorite
      vegetables

   ½ lime (optional)

1. Rinse kombu under cold water and place it in a 6-quart saucepan with about 6½ cups water. Bring to a boil.

2. As the kombu water is coming to a boil, combine the soy sauce and mirin in a small saucepan, then place over high heat. When this boils, add the sweetener and boil for 30 more seconds. Remove from heat, transfer to a glass bowl, and cover with a damp kitchen towel.

3. Pour 1 cup boiling water on the shiitake mushrooms and let them sit for 15 minutes. Drain the water through a strainer into the kombu water, and gently squeeze the mushrooms to remove any excess liquid. Slice them very thin.

4. Heat oil in the skillet, add 1 tablespoon garlic, and when it has begun to turn color, add the mushrooms. Sauté them for a few minutes on each side.

5. When the kombu water is boiling, keep at a boil for about 5 minutes, then remove the kombu and add the noodles, the remaining tablespoon of garlic, and the ginger. Cook, stirring often, for 5 minutes. Continue to cook until the noodles are al dente.

6. Remove the soup from the heat and stir in the soy sauce mixture, the tofu, the mushrooms, the scallions, and any of the optional vegetables you wish to add. Cover and set aside for 1 minute. Squeeze in the lime juice (optional).

MOCK CHILI CON QUESO

Serves 8

This is from Annette Spaniel, an animal activist in Dallas, Texas. Luscious. Meat eaters love it. I quadrupled the recipe and served it to forty youth one winter with great success.

Queso Spread

One 15-ounce can Great Northern beans (about 1½ cups), rinsed well and drained

½ cup pimento pieces, drained

6 tablespoons nutritional yeast flakes

3 tablespoons fresh lemon juice

2–3 tablespoons tahini

½ teaspoon onion granules

½ teaspoon prepared yellow mustard

½ teaspoon salt

½ teaspoon garlic powder

One or two 10-ounce cans diced tomatoes and chilies (use Ro·Tel brand, if available in your area), drained

1. Place all the ingredients except canned tomatoes in a blender, and process until completely smooth.
2. Stir in a can or more of the tomatoes, depending on taste. (Drain first, reserve the liquid to add later in case you want to thin the chili); choose the spicy variety if you want spicy chili.
3. Put aside while you prepare the chili.

Chili

3½ cups water

1 6.4-ounce box Fantastic Foods vegetarian chili (or equivalent amount of a bulk or packaged vegetarian chili mix)

Two 15-ounce cans (2½ cups) kidney, pinto, or red beans
  (drained and rinsed) or 2½ cups cooked beans

One 14-ounce can diced or stewed tomatoes

1. Bring water to a boil. Add the chili mix and stir well. Add beans and
   tomatoes.
2. Reduce heat and simmer, uncovered, for 25 minutes. Stir often,
   because the chili has a tendency to stick to the bottom of the pan.
3. Fold the "queso" spread into the cooked chili and heat through.

Best if prepared a day ahead of time so that the flavors can blend.

MISO MAYONNAISE

Makes about ²/₃ cup

Miso mayonnaise is a tasty alternative to regular mayonnaise. It makes a great dip for vegetables, or a spread for bread. Who needs an expensive store-bought version when this one is so easy and quick?

½ shallot
1½ tablespoons apple cider vinegar
1½ tablespoons tamari/soy sauce
3 tablespoons chickpea miso
½ cup canola oil

Blend together in a blender until smooth. Refrigerate when not using.

PESTO

Makes approximately 1¹/₂ cups

Serve with your favorite pasta, on toasted Italian bread as an appetizer, as a layer in lasagna, or on pizza.

2 cups lightly packed fresh basil
3 medium-large garlic cloves
1 cup toasted walnuts, pine nuts, or pecans
1–1¹/₂ tablespoons red miso
²/₃ cup olive oil
Pinch salt

1. Put all ingredients except salt in food processor. Process until creamy, but not completely smooth. Salt to taste.
2. Just before serving with pasta, add a little hot pasta water to awaken the flavors.

BARBECUE SAUCE

Makes 4 servings

A tasty sauce. Serve with Golden Fried Tofu.

 1 onion, chopped
 1 large clove garlic, chopped
 ¼ cup apple butter
 1 slight teaspoon chili paste
 ¼ cup fresh lemon juice
 1 tablespoon corn oil
 1 tablespoon vegetarian Worcestershire sauce
 ½ cup tomato sauce
 2 teaspoons dry mustard
 1 tablespoon Sucanat or other sweetener
 ½ teaspoon salt
 1 recipe Golden Fried Tofu (page 253)

1. Place onion and garlic in a food processor or blender, and pulse until finely chopped.
2. Add apple butter, chili paste, and lemon juice. Process again, so that the mixture is well blended.
3. Add the oil, Worcestershire sauce, tomato sauce, mustard, sweetener, and salt, and process until mixed. Transfer sauce to a saucepan and simmer for 30 minutes, stirring occasionally.
4. Prepare Golden Fried Tofu. When it is ready, add the barbecue sauce to the saucepan to coat the tofu well, and simmer the tofu in the sauce for about 15 minutes.
5. Dish the remaining sauce into a serving bowl. Serve with rice and pass the sauce.

RICH SHIITAKE MUSHROOM SAUCE

Yield: two cups

Serve this mushroomy sauce over pasta, tofu, or vegetables.

12 dried shiitake mushrooms, mixed sizes
4 tablespoons tamari
1 tablespoon sherry
1 teaspoon Sucanat or other sweetener
$\frac{1}{4}$ teaspoon salt
2–3 tablespoons oil
1 tablespoon cornstarch

1. Soak dried mushrooms in at least 2 cups hot water for 15 minutes. Reserve the soaking liquid.
2. Slice the large mushrooms; leave small mushrooms whole.
3. Combine tamari, sherry, sweetener, and salt.
4. Heat oil. Add mushrooms and stir-fry 2 minutes. Stir in tamari-sherry mixture to blend.
5. Add mushroom liquid and heat quickly. Then cook, covered, about 10 minutes over medium heat.
6. Blend cornstarch and 1 tablespoon cold water to make a paste. Then stir into the sauce to thicken. Keep warm till serving.

HOT PEANUT SAUCE

Yield: 5–6 servings

You can pour this sauce over tofu, steamed or stir-fried veggies, noodles, or rice.

- 3 tablespoons peanut butter
- 2 tablespoons roasted sesame oil
- 2 tablespoons soy sauce
- 2 tablespoons sherry
- 2 tablespoons Sucanat or other sweetener
- 3 tablespoons vegetable broth
- 1 tablespoon hoisin sauce
- 2 tablespoons tomato sauce
- 1 teaspoon chili sauce or ½ teaspoon chili oil

1. Mix all ingredients together in a saucepan.
2. Over low heat, warm the sauce for 3 to 5 minutes, stirring frequently. Pour over the food of your choice.

MARY'S MUSHROOM SAUCE

Serves 4 to 6

My good friend Mary Hunt directed me to this recipe found in Anna Thomas's classic, *The Vegetarian Epicure*. I have revised it, reducing the amount of fat she recommended and the sugar as well. I served this over toast to some very firmly committed meat eaters. They enjoyed it immensely, but felt that at $^1/_3$ cup sugar, it was still too sweet. Others might like it that way. You should experiment with it and see what you prefer.

$1^1/_2$ pound fresh mushrooms
$^1/_4$ cup light oil/vegan margarine (I use a combination)
1 onion, peeled and chopped
2 tablespoons Dijon mustard
$^1/_4$ to $^1/_3$ cup brown sugar or Sucanat
2 tablespoons vegetarian Worcestershire sauce
$^3/_4$ cup mellow red wine
Freshly ground black pepper
Seasoned salt
Dash of Tabasco

1. Clean the mushrooms and cut each one in half, unless they are very small. In a large saucepan, warm the oil/margarine and sauté the onion until transparent.
2. Mix together the mustard, sweetener, and Worcestershire sauce into a smooth paste. Add the wine, and season with black pepper and a little seasoned salt. Stir well.
3. When the onion is transparent, add the mushrooms to the pan. Sauté a few minutes. Stir often. When the mushrooms begin to brown and reduce in size, add the sauce.
4. Simmer the mixture for 45 minutes over medium-low to medium heat. The mushrooms will darken, and the sauce will thicken and reduce.

SQUASH SAUCE

Serves 5 to 6, unless they are teenagers

A vegan in Cincinnati discovered that squash is a great thickener for pasta sauces and a delightful way to create a comfort food close to macaroni and cheese. She pressed a recipe into my hand when I spoke there. I encountered a recipe in Ken Haedrich's *Feeding the Healthy Vegetarian Family* that works with this insight as well. It is incredibly like macaroni and cheese, yet it is dairyless. This sauce is an adaptation of Haedrich's recipe.

3 tablespoons olive oil

1 large onion, chopped

1 or 2 cloves garlic, minced

1½ cups canned or frozen squash

1½ cups plain unsweetened soy milk

3 tablespoons nutritional yeast flakes

1 teaspoon Dijon mustard (My family doesn't like mustard in this; some would probably be happy with 2 teaspoons.)

1 teaspoon salt

Freshly ground pepper

2 to 3 tablespoons chopped fresh parsley

1. If using frozen squash, defrost it.

2. In a large nonstick skillet, heat 2 tablespoons of the olive oil. Stir in the onion and sauté over medium heat for 8 to 10 minutes. Add the garlic, stir for half a minute, then remove from the heat.

3. Put the squash, soy milk, nutritional yeast flakes, mustard, remaining tablespoon of olive oil, onions, and salt in a blender or use an immersion blender. Puree until the mixture is smooth. Pour it into the skillet that cooked the onions. Heat the sauce, stirring, until it bubbles. Add pepper. Garnish with parsley and serve over cooked macaroni.

SIDE DISHES AND SALADS

COMFORTING MASHED POTATOES

Makes 4 servings

2 pounds Russet or Idaho potatoes, scrubbed and quartered
   (If organic, leave the skins on.)
1 32-ounce box of Imagine No-Chicken Broth
8 cloves garlic, peeled
1 cup plain soy milk
1 cup soy cream (I use Silk.)
4 tablespoons vegan margarine
Salt and freshly ground pepper to taste
1/2 cup minced Italian parsley (not curly, but flat-leafed)
   (optional)

1. Boil the quartered potatoes uncovered in a large pot with broth until tender, about twenty minutes. Remove the potatoes from the broth, but do not discard the broth.
2. While the potatoes are cooking, put garlic cloves, soy milk, and soy cream into a medium saucepan. Simmer uncovered over low heat until garlic is tender, about 15 minutes. Remove garlic cloves.
3. Combine the potatoes and the simmered milk-cream mixture in a large bowl with margarine and mash with a potato masher. If it needs thinning, add some of the broth. Season with salt and pepper to taste. Add minced parsley if you wish, and serve.

NUTTY CABBAGE SALAD

Serves 8

The salad I made for my family that kept them coming back for more. (See page 196.) I have reduced the amount of oil that the original recipe called for, but I have also seen versions of this recipe that use only the sesame oil and not the canola. Experiment with the quantity according to your taste buds.

- 5 cups shredded cabbage
- 1 leaf red cabbage, shredded
- 2 carrots, shredded
- 8 scallions, sliced
- $\frac{1}{2}$ cup slivered almonds
- $\frac{1}{4}$ cup sesame seeds
- 1 tablespoon vegan margarine
- 1 teaspoon pepper
- 2 packages Ramen noodles. Use the noodles, uncooked, and discard the flavor packet.

Dressing

- 6 tablespoons rice vinegar
- 3 tablespoons Sucanat or other sweetener
- $\frac{1}{3}$–$\frac{1}{2}$ cup canola oil
- 1 tablespoon toasted sesame oil
- 2 teaspoons salt
- 1 teaspoon pepper
- $\frac{1}{4}$ cup fresh cilantro (optional)

1. Brown the almonds and sesame seeds in the margarine. Set aside.
2. Shred cabbage and carrots.
3. Make the dressing.
4. Crumble the noodles, or put them in a plastic bag and smash them with a hammer.
5. Just before serving, pour dressing over the vegetables until they are moistened. Reserve the rest of the dressing. Add the crumbled noodles. Toss the salad, then sprinkle with the cooled almonds and sesame seeds, and, if desired, the cilantro.

POTSTICKERS

Serves 4

Vegetarian potstickers (Chinese dumplings) are available in Asian food stores and in some natural food stores as well. My children, Doug and Ben, love these dumplings dipped in the dressing.

1 pound frozen vegetarian potstickers
1 tablespoon vegetable oil (optional)

1. Arrange frozen potstickers in a single layer in a 10- to 12-inch nonstick frying pan, and add ⅔ cup water. Cover and bring to a boil over high heat.
2. Once the water has begun to boil, reduce the heat and simmer until the liquid cooks away and potstickers begin to brown, (about 12 to 15 minutes). Keep covered, but check the bottom of the potstickers. When the water has cooked away, if you like more crispness to the dumplings, add 1 tablespoon oil to the pan, and gently lift each dumpling up so that the oil dodges underneath them.

Dressing for Potstickers

$1/4$ cup hoisin sauce

2 tablespoons lemon juice

1 teaspoon toasted sesame oil

1 teaspoon Sucanat or other sweetener

1 teaspoon minced fresh ginger

1 clove garlic, minced

Potsticker Salad

I prefer the dumplings in a salad.

Nine ounces salad mix or 8 cups fresh greens

One $7^{1}/_{4}$-ounce jar peeled roasted red or yellow peppers,
drained, or 2 roasted peppers, sliced into thin strips

As the dumplings cook, prepare the salad and make the dressing. Toss the greens with the dressing, spoon salad onto 4 plates, and top with equal portions of red peppers and hot potstickers.

Golden Tomato Tart

Serves 6

One makes this simply for the sheer joy of its appearance and taste. There are much easier things to do with tomatoes. This is for a summer day when you want to celebrate the glorious abundance of tomatoes. You can take it on a picnic, use it as an appetizer, or arrange a meal around it. I have adapted it from a recipe developed by Viana La Place that appears in her book *Verdura: Vegetables Italian Style.*

> 4 tablespoons olive oil
>
> 1 clove garlic, peeled and crushed into a paste
>
> 7 tomatoes (La Place uses Roma tomatoes, but I have also used regular tomatoes.)
>
> 1 sheet puff pastry dough, 12 by 12 inches (follow instructions on box for rolling out)
>
> 1 teaspoon Ener-G Egg Replacer or 1 teaspoon cornstarch beaten in 2 tablespoons water
>
> 14 basil leaves, sliced thin
>
> Salt and freshly ground black pepper
>
> 1/4 cup toasted pine nuts

1. Combine the olive oil and garlic in a small bowl and set aside.
2. Core, slice, and seed the tomatoes. Seeding can be tedious, but unless you seed the tomatoes, your puff pastry will become drenched in unnecessary tomato juice. Drain the seeded tomatoes on paper towels.
3. Arrange the puff pastry dough on a baking sheet. Cut 1/2-inch strips from all four sides of the dough. Brush reconstituted Egg Replacer or cornstarch mixture on the edges of the square of dough and arrange the strips on the top of the edges. Prick the bottom of the dough with a fork. Refrigerate for about one hour.

4. Preheat the oven to 400 degrees.

5. Bake the dough for 10 minutes or until it has risen and turns slightly golden.

6. Brush with 2 tablespoons of the garlic-infused olive oil and distribute half of the basil over it.

7. Season with salt and pepper to taste.

8. Arrange the tomato slices over the top in an overlapping pattern.

9. Top with the remaining garlic-infused olive oil.

10. Bake for 10 minutes, or until the pastry is golden, and the tomatoes have softened, but are still intact. Cool slightly.

11. Sprinkle the pine nuts and the remaining basil over the tart.

BEN'S FAVORITE SALAD DRESSING

Yield: ¹/₂ cup

2 tablespoons white miso, thinned with a little warm water

¹/₃ cup olive oil

¹/₄ cup balsamic vinegar

2 cloves garlic, minced

¹/₂ teaspoon oregano

2 teaspoons raspberry jam

Mix together and serve over your favorite salad mix.

PAPAYA SEED DRESSING

Yield: About 2 cups / 8 servings

This dressing is adapted from Bonnie Mandoe's *Vegetarian Nights.* It gets a zip from the papaya seeds. Extremely tasty, it also provides the gratification of being able to use a part of the papaya that is so often discarded. Besides putting it on salads, I have sprinkled it over vegetable pizzas for pizzazz.

$\frac{1}{4}$ cup chopped onion

1 large clove garlic, minced

2 tablespoons Dijon mustard

3 tablespoons brown rice syrup

$1\frac{1}{2}$ teaspoons salt

$\frac{1}{4}$ cup olive oil

$\frac{3}{4}$ cup canola or sunflower oil

$\frac{1}{4}$ cup rice vinegar

1 tablespoon balsamic vinegar

$\frac{1}{2}$ teaspoon dried basil leaves

$\frac{1}{2}$ teaspoon dried oregano leaves

$\frac{1}{4}$ cup water

2 tablespoons papaya seeds

1. Put all the ingredients into a blender and blend for about a minute to a minute and a half. The papaya seeds should be fragmented by the blades. This is a creamy dressing with speckles of papaya seeds.
2. Chill the dressing and serve.

BAKED GOODS AND DESSERTS

BASIC MUFFINS

Yield: 12 muffins

Many children love to fix baked goods. If they are preschool age (and you have a clean floor), you can perform step 2 on the floor. It is the perfect mixing platform for children.

 $\frac{1}{2}$ cup soft tofu

 6 teaspoons Ener-G Egg Replacer

 $\frac{1}{2}$ cup sunflower or safflower oil

 $\frac{3}{4}$ cup maple syrup or $1\frac{1}{4}$ cup FruitSource

 1 ripe banana

 $1\frac{1}{2}$ cups whole wheat pastry flour

 $\frac{1}{2}$ cup soy flour

 $\frac{1}{4}$ cup oat bran (make your own with oats pulverized in a blender)

 Dash salt

 $2\frac{1}{2}$ teaspoons baking powder

 $\frac{1}{2}$ teaspoon grated nutmeg

 1 teaspoon ground cinnamon

Mango Muffins

 2 mangoes, cut into $\frac{1}{2}$-inch cubes

Carob Muffins

 $\frac{1}{8}$ to $\frac{1}{4}$ cup soy milk for thinning

 $\frac{1}{2}$ to $\frac{3}{4}$ cup carob chips

 1 tablespoon vanilla

Lemon Poppyseed Muffins

 3 tablespoons poppyseeds
 Zest of 3 small lemons, minced
 $\frac{1}{3}$ to $\frac{1}{2}$ cup lemon juice

1. Preheat oven to 400 degrees. Oil 12 muffin cups. Put tofu, Egg Replacer, oil, sweetener, and banana into a food processor. If you are making lemon poppyseed muffins, add the lemon juice; if you are making carob muffins, add the soy milk and vanilla. Cream together.

2. Combine the flours, oat bran, salt, baking powder, nutmeg, and cinnamon in a large bowl. Make a well in the center of the dry ingredients and add the banana mixture. Using a spatula, quickly fold the wet ingredients into the dry. Don't overmix.

3. Depending on which muffins you are making, add either the mango, carob chips, or lemon zest and poppyseeds. Fold them into the batter.

4. Spoon batter into muffin cups. Fill each cup about $\frac{2}{3}$ full. Bake for 25 to 30 minutes. The muffins should be lightly browned. A toothpick inserted into the center of the muffin should come out clean. Cool briefly.

THE BEST SCONE RECIPE IN THE WORLD

Makes 16 large scones

This scone recipe is hands down the most popular food that emerges from our kitchen. It can be used as an after-school snack, a morning breakfast treat, or a dessert. Because it uses so much less sugar and fat than chocolate chip cookies, it is a healthier way to treat anyone to chocolate desserts. And its biggest attraction is that, if you have the ingredients on hand, it can be whipped up in minutes. Mixing baking soda and vinegar causes a volcanolike explosion in elementary school science demonstrations; they perform the same function here, giving the scones a light and airy texture.

I have adapted this recipe from a Lorna Sass recipe that I found in her book *Short-Cut Vegetarian*.

Serve the scones warm, or soon thereafter.

1 tablespoon apple cider vinegar

Approximately 1 cup soy milk

1 1/2 cups unbleached all-purpose flour

1 1/2 cups spelt flour or whole wheat pastry flour

3/8 cup Sucanat or other sweetener

3 teaspoons baking powder

3/4 teaspoon baking soda

3/4 teaspoon salt

1/2 cup Spectrum Spread

3 teaspoons vanilla extract

Chocolate Chip Scones

1 cup chocolate chips (or more!)

My Favorite Nonchocolate Scones

$\frac{1}{2}$ cup toasted walnuts, coarsely chopped

$\frac{1}{2}$ cup dried cherries

$\frac{1}{2}$ cup carob chips

1. Place the rack in the middle of the oven.
2. Preheat the oven to 425 degrees. Lightly mist a nonstick cookie sheet with vegetable oil cooking spray or line with parchment paper.
3. Put apple cider vinegar into a 1-cup measuring cup and add enough soy milk to bring it level to 1 cup. Set aside. The mixture will be clabbered, like buttermilk.
4. In a large mixing bowl, mix together the dry ingredients. Add the Spectrum Spread to the dry ingredients, and cut it in using a pastry blender or two knives or your fingers. The mixture will be crumbly now.
5. Add the chocolate chips or the walnut-cherry-carob mixture to the bowl and mix them in.
6. Add the vanilla to the vinegar and soy milk mixture and pour almost all of this mixture into the dry ingredients.
7. Stir quickly with a spatula only until the mixture forms a soft dough. You don't want a gooey mess, so add more soy milk only if the dough still seems crumbly rather than doughy.
8. Turn the dough onto the cookie sheet in 4 equal parts. Shape each part into a thick circle about 5–7 inches in diameter. Using a sharp knife, score the top of each circle, dividing it into quarters. (For smaller scones, divide the dough into 6 wedges.)
9. Bake for 12 minutes. A toothpick stuck into the middle of each scone should come out clean, and the bottoms will be lightly browned. Don't let them bake too long, but they may need a few more minutes. Transfer them to a wire rack and enjoy.

SOY "BUTTERMILK" BISCUITS

Yield: 10 to 12 biscuits

Easy, quick, and tasty. Great with soups or jam.

> Scant 1 tablespoon apple cider vinegar
> $^3/_4$ cup soy milk
> 1 cup white flour
> $1^1/_4$ cups spelt or pastry flour
> 1 tablespoon baking powder
> $^1/_4$ teaspoon baking soda
> $^1/_2$ teaspoon salt
> $^1/_3$ cup safflower oil

1. Preheat the oven to 450 degrees.
2. Measure the vinegar and place into a measuring cup. Pour the soy milk in until it measures $^3/_4$ cup. Leave to curdle while combining the dry ingredients.
3. Sift the flours, baking powder, baking soda, and salt together into a mixing bowl. Make a well in the center, and pour in the oil and soy "buttermilk." Use a fork to combine, but do not overmix. Mix quickly and conservatively.
4. Lightly flour a surface, and turn the dough onto it. Knead it gently a few times. Pat the dough until it is about $^1/_2$ inch thick. Using a biscuit cutter or a glass, cut the dough into 10 to 12 biscuits. Place them so that they touch each other on an ungreased baking sheet.
5. Bake for 10 to 12 minutes, until golden brown. Serve immediately.

CAROB CAKE

Yield: a 2–layer cake

This is a very light and moist cake. I adapted it from the Bloodroot Collective's *Perennial Political Palate*. For several years now, the women of Bloodroot have been developing delicious uses for sourdough cultures.

Dry Ingredients

7 tablespoons carob

$1\frac{1}{2}$ cups Sucanat or other sweetener

3 cups unbleached white flour

2 teaspoons baking soda

$\frac{1}{2}$ teaspoon salt

$\frac{1}{2}$ teaspoon each cinnamon and nutmeg, freshly grated if possible

1 tablespoon powdered coffee substitute

Wet Ingredients

1 cup awakened sourdough culture (Follow directions on pages 231–232.)

1 cup vanilla or carob soy milk

$\frac{2}{3}$ cup water

2 tablespoons vinegar

1 cup oil

1 tablespoon vanilla

2 tablespoons maple syrup

1. Lightly oil two 9-inch round pans. Line with parchment paper.
2. Preheat oven to 350 degrees.
3. Sift dry ingredients together. Set aside.

4. In a different bowl, combine wet ingredients.

5. Use a wooden spoon to mix wet and dry ingredients together with as few strokes as possible.

6. Divide the batter between the two pans and place in preheated oven. Bake for 25 to 30 minutes, or until just done. Cake will have pulled away from the edges of the pan. A toothpick inserted in the middle should come out clean.

7. Cool five minutes on a rack, then turn out onto the rack. Peel off and discard parchment paper. Let cool thoroughly.

Variation: You can make a light and delicious spice cake by omitting the carob powder and coffee and adding $1/4$ teaspoon cloves with the cinnamon and nutmeg.

Frosting

1 cup Sucanat

$1/4$ cup water

3 tablespoons carob

1 tablespoon coffee substitute (see About Ingredients)

2 teaspoons vanilla

$1/2$ teaspoon each cinnamon and nutmeg

3 ounces in weight vegan margarine, softened to room temperature

1. Stir the Sucanat and water over low heat until the sweetener has melted.

2. Bring the mixture to a boil and remove from heat.

3. Beat in the carob, coffee substitute, vanilla, and spices.

4. Stir frequently as it cools. When it is room temperature—and not before—gradually add the margarine. Frost cake. Enjoy!

OATMEAL CHOCOLATE CHIP COOKIES

Yield: 18–24 cookies (allowing for a little nibbling on the dough)

Oil for cookie sheet

³/₄ cup unbleached flour or spelt flour

¹/₂ teaspoon baking soda

¹/₂ teaspoon baking powder

¹/₂ teaspoon sea salt

¹/₃ cup soft tofu

¹/₃ cup canola or safflower oil

¹/₄ cup FruitSource or concentrated fruit juice

1 tablespoon vanilla extract

¹/₂ cup Sucanat or other sweetener

¹/₄ cup brown rice syrup

2 cups rolled oats (quick oats, if available)

2 cups vegan semisweet chocolate chips or carob chips

1 cup chopped toasted walnuts (optional)

1. Preheat oven to 350 degrees. Oil a cookie sheet with canola oil or a cooking spray.
2. In a small bowl blend the flour, baking soda, baking powder, and salt. Set aside.
3. Wash the tofu under running water, then thoroughly whip it in your mixer until creamy. At low speed add the oil, FruitSource, vanilla, and Sucanat. Mix until the Sucanat is somewhat dissolved, then add the brown rice syrup. Mix for another minute until the sweeteners are well blended.
4. Add the oats and the flour mixture. Blend thoroughly, about 2 minutes. Fold in the chips and, if desired, the walnuts.

5. Drop a generous spoonful of dough on the cookie sheet. Gently flatten the dough with your spoon, as the cookies will not spread during baking.

6. Bake for 13–15 minutes. For a soft cookie, cool the cookies on a flat surface like your countertop. For a crunchier texture, cool on a metal cooling rack.

STRAWBERRY SHORTCAKE

6–8 servings

This is a flavored shortcake, and while it can be eaten as a bread it goes tremendously with fresh strawberries. You need saffron threads for the recipe, but if you cannot get them, you can omit them and the shortcake will still be tasty. I have adapted this recipe from a bread that I found in Miriam Kasin Hospodar's *Heaven's Banquet.* My partner, Bruce, suggested using it as a shortcake for strawberries.

    1 quart strawberries

Clean, hull, and slice strawberries. Sprinkle a little Sucanat on them and refrigerate.

Shortcake

¼ teaspoon very loosely packed saffron threads (Don't
   push them in too much!)

¼ cup hot water

¼ cup vegan margarine (preferably Spectrum Spread)

1 cup Sucanat or other sweetener

1 cup Tofutti Better Than Sour Cream (In a pinch you can
   use soy yogurt.)

1 tablespoon finely grated lemon zest

¼ cup lemon juice

½ cup soy milk

1¼ cups unbleached white flour

1¼ cups pastry flour or spelt flour

2 tablespoons arrowroot or cornstarch

2 teaspoons baking powder

½ teaspoon baking soda

1 teaspoon salt

1 cup sliced almonds, toasted

1. Preheat the oven to 350 degrees.
2. Oil and lightly flour a 9 × 5 × 3-inch loaf pan, or 3 small loaf pans.
3. With your fingers, crumble the saffron threads into a small bowl. Add the hot water, stir, and put aside while you prepare the other ingredients.
4. Cream the vegan margarine and Sucanat together. Add Better Than Sour Cream, lemon zest, lemon juice, and soy milk, and beat together until smooth. Add the saffron water.
5. Mix the flours, arrowroot or cornstarch, salt, baking powder, and soda together.
6. Make a well in the dry ingredients and add the wet ingredients. Mix only until all the ingredients are blended. Add the almonds. If the shortcake looks too dry, add just a little more soy milk.

7. Spoon the batter into the loaf pan (or pans). Bake for about 40 to 50 minutes for the large pan, or about 30 to 40 minutes for the smaller ones. Be sure to check with a toothpick before removing from the oven.

GINGERBREAD

Makes one 9 × 9-inch cake

One last recipe from Jennifer Raymond. In *The Peaceful Palate,* she writes: "This gingerbread contains no animal ingredients and no added fat, yet it is moist and delicious. Try serving it with hot applesauce for a real treat." It is a great recipe, and will confirm your magician-like skills to your meat-eating friends and family.

$^1\!/_2$ cup raisins

$^1\!/_2$ cup pitted dates, chopped

$1^3\!/_4$ cups water

$^3\!/_4$ cup raw sugar or other sweetener

$^1\!/_2$ teaspoon salt

2 teaspoons cinnamon

1 teaspoon ginger

$^3\!/_4$ teaspoon nutmeg

$^1\!/_4$ teaspoon cloves

2 cups flour (Jennifer uses whole wheat pastry flour.)

1 teaspoon baking soda

1 teaspoon baking powder

1. Preheat oven to 350 degrees.
2. Combine dried fruits, water, sugar, and spices in a large saucepan and bring to a boil. Continue boiling for 2 minutes, then remove from heat and cool completely.
3. When fruit mixture is cool, mix in dry ingredients. Spread into a greased 9 × 9-inch pan and bake for 30 minutes or until a toothpick inserted into the center comes out clean.

QUICK "DO NOT STIR" BLACKBERRY COBBLER

Serves 4 to 6

This is a fun and quick dessert that is splendidly rich and delicious. I like using spelt flour for this recipe instead of whole wheat pastry flour, because it is light. But pastry flour can be substituted. Remember: don't stir it!

You can substitute other fresh fruits, but somehow blackberries are perfect for this. Frozen fruits work as well. Though southern tradition suggests that canned fruits might also be used, I have found them the least successful.

$^1/_4$ cup vegan margarine

$^3/_4$ cup Sucanat (plus extra for sprinkling over berries) or other sweetener

1 cup spelt flour

3 teaspoons baking powder

1 cup vanilla soy milk (For a real treat use a soy cream like Silk.)

4 cups fresh blackberries, drained

$^1/_2$ teaspoon cinnamon

$^1/_2$ teaspoon nutmeg

1. Preheat oven to 350 degrees.
2. Melt vegan margarine over low heat in an oblong rectangular baking dish.
3. In a separate bowl, combine Sucanat, flour, and baking powder. Whisk in the soy milk or soy cream to make a batter.
4. Pour the batter over the melted margarine. Do not stir.
5. Top with the blackberries. Do not stir them into the batter. Sprinkle a little Sucanat over the fruit and then sprinkle the cinnamon and nutmeg on. Again, do not stir.
6. Bake for 40 to 50 minutes, until the top is golden brown. The batter will rise through the blackberries and form a delicate and delicious crust. You can also use a toothpick test (it should come out clean) to make sure the batter is cooked. This is supposed to make 4 to 6 servings, but one night three of us unabashedly devoured the entire cobbler.

CHOCOLATE CREAM PIE

Serves 6 to 8

We take this to church socials, feed it to hungry teens, and use it for birthday celebrations. No one can believe it has tofu in it.

  1½ to 2 cups vegan chocolate chips
  2 boxes firm silken tofu
  1 tablespoon vanilla
  1 large graham cracker crust
  Fruit (optional)

1. Melt the chocolate chips over low heat, stirring constantly.
2. Put the silken tofu in a food processor and puree.
3. Add the melted chocolate chips and process until smooth.
4. Add the vanilla and process.
5. Pour into the crust and refrigerate for a couple of hours.
6. Add strawberries, kiwi, or other fruits to the top if you wish, but no fruits are necessary for this delicious dessert.

About Ingredients and Products

Brown rice syrup is a liquid sweetener derived from brown rice. It is a delicious alternative to honey and it works effectively in baked goods. (See also FruitSource.) It is less sweet than honey, but if you use it as a honey substitute you might find that you do not have to increase the amount of brown rice syrup because the depth of its flavor adequately compensates for the cloying sweetness of honey. When using liquid sweeteners like brown rice syrup, measure your oil first and then the measuring cup will have a coating that will allow the syrup to slide out.

"Chicken flavored" vegetarian stock powder is available at many natural food stores. It can be used to make "unchicken" noodle soups, as an alternative flavoring for soup recipes that call for "chicken stock." I also sprinkle some in a little water and cook broccoli in it until the water has evaporated and add a teaspoon or so to cream sauces.

Coffee substitutes are usually made from a combination of roasted barley, malt, chicory, rye, and beet root. Other ingredients may be figs, carob, almonds, and dates. They contain no caffeine. In baked goods they can be used with carob to provide an alternative to chocolate. The coffee substitute deepens the flavor, and is suggestive of mocha. I have used Instant/Sipp Natural Coffee Substitute, but I have also encountered exotic offerings such as Teeccino Almond Amaretto Caffeine-Free Herbal Coffee.

Ener-G Egg Replacer is the brand name of a powder that one can use in the place of eggs. Its ingredients include potato starch, tapioca flour, dairy-free calcium lactate, calcium carbonate, citric acid, and carbohydrate gum. Mixing $1\frac{1}{2}$ teaspoons egg replacer with two tablespoons water creates the equivalent of one egg. One can also use bananas, soft tofu, arrowroot powder, or cornstarch as a binder in baked goods.

FruitSource is a liquid sweetener and fat replacer made from organic brown rice syrup and grape juice concentrate. It has the consistency of honey, an appealing amber color, and a wonderful aroma to it. Because of the grape juice, its sweetness is stronger than that of brown rice syrup.

Imagine Natural Garden Vegetable Soups are a line of soups from Imagine Foods. Their "no-chicken broth" is a convenient base for many soups, such as the African Bean Soup.

Kombu is a stiff, black sea vegetable, sold in almost footlong strips. It provides an instant stock when boiled for several minutes.

Mirin is a sweet Japanese cooking wine made from sweet rice. The best-quality mirin is made from sweet rice, rice koji, and water with no added sugar, alcohol, or fermenting agents.

Miso is a fermented soybean paste that adds flavor to sauces and soups. Some misos are made solely from soybeans and salt. Others are made from soybeans, salt, and a grain such as rice or barley, or legumes such as chickpeas. It is a fine source of high-quality protein. It provides a salty flavor, and can mimic, at times, Parmesan cheese in some recipes (see, for instance, the pesto recipe). Avoid boiling miso once you have added it to a dish because intense heat will destroy its healthful enzymes. Keep refrigerated. Miso is found in health food stores, natural food stores, and Asian food stores.

Nutritional Yeast Flakes refers to Red Star formula (T6635+) nutritional yeast flakes. Do not confuse it with brewer's yeast. Yeast flakes provide a "cheesy" flavor to foods.

Olive oil. When I say olive oil, I mean extra-virgin, cold-pressed olive oil.

Puff pastry. Pepperidge Farm makes a frozen vegan puff pastry, which I have used in the recipes. Follow the instructions for defrosting the puff pastry, and use according to the recipe.

Spectrum Spread is a nonhydrogenated vegetable shortening that is used instead of butter. I always keep some on hand for making scones and cobblers. Available in natural food stores.

Sucanat is a sugarcane sweetener. It is my favorite dry sweetener because I like the way it performs in recipes.

Sucanat stands for SUgar CAne NATural. It is an evaporated sugar-cane juice. It contains more minerals, trace elements, and vitamins than table sugar. I like it because it has an inviting taste and adds a depth of flavor to baked goods and other items that call for a dry sweetener. You can substitute it for refined sugar, one cup for one cup.

Tamari soy sauce is a fermented soy sauce made from soybeans, salt, water, and a starter called *koji*. It is nothing like commercial soy sauce, which is indebted to caramel for its dark brown color and to corn syrup for its sweetness. Tamari soy sauce's fermentation occurs through the introduction of a soybean starter. I like tamari's taste, which seems fuller, and it contains more amino acids. If you cannot eat fermented foods, you may enjoy the tasty alternative of Bragg Liquid Aminos.

Tofu is an inexpensive, versatile, high-quality protein, cholesterol-free, rich-in-calcium, soybean product. It is made by a process similar to making cheese: soy milk is coagulated, drained, and then the curds are pressed into a cake. (Home tofu kits are now available.) The fear of tofu is due, in part, to its blandness. In fact, its "blandness" is what makes it so versatile because of its ability to absorb a variety of flavors. Tofu is labeled according to its water content. The less water it contains, the firmer the tofu is and the more likely it is to hold its shape in cooking. Regular tofu is packed in water, and usually found in plastic tubs in the refrigerator section of a health foods store, as well as the produce section of more and more supermarkets. Keep it refrigerated. Silken tofu is creamy, smooth, and available in aseptic boxes that do not require refrigeration. If you are frying or baking tofu, use regular tofu. If you are using tofu in baked goods, creamy soups, puddings, or cream pies, use silken tofu.

Tofutti products are a line of products that contain no dairy, no cholesterol, no lactose, no butterfat, yet are amazingly similar to their dairy equivalent. Among the offerings from Tofutti are "Better Than Sour Cream Sour Supreme" and "Better Than Cream Cheese." They are remarkable substitutes for almost any recipe that calls for sour cream or cream cheese. For many years, one of my sons took for his school lunch a bagel with Better Than Cream Cheese spread on it. A tablespoon of

Sour Supreme is great added to one's gazpacho soup bowl or on tortillas.

TVP is texturized vegetable protein. It is made from soy flour. After the soybean oil has been extracted, cooked under pressure, extruded, and dried the result is a dense textured food that is chewy and "meatlike." It is sold in granules, flakes, chunks, or slices. When rehydrated the granules resemble ground "beef" and the chunks have the texture and appearance of chunks of "meat." Especially, when cooked in certain ways, it is often mistaken for meat and it can be substituted for meat, such as "hamburger," in recipes like "sloppy joes." TVP is an excellent source of protein and fiber, and has zero cholesterol. The initials are the registered trademark of the Archer Daniels Midland Company.

Udon noodles are a flat Japanese wheat noodle similar to fettuccine. Light in color, they have a delightful, chewy texture.

Vegan margarine. Many margarines have some dairy products in them. Vegan margarines do not. An example is Earth Balance Natural Buttery Spread. Some brands, such as this one, are not hydrogenated and have no trans fatty acids. At times I recommend "Spectrum Spread," which is also nonhydrogenated. It makes baked goods like cobblers and scones very delicious.

Vegetarian Worcestershire sauce may be carried by your local natural foods store, or you can order it from PANGEA (1-800-340-1200, 2381 Lewis Avenue, Rockville, MD 20852), or order on-line at www.veg-anstore.com.

Wheat Meat or Chicken Style Wheat Meat are two of the brands of seitan now available. Seitan is made from wheat gluten and is a good protein alternative for those who have soy allergies. Like tofu, it is versatile in its uses. Seitan is a high protein, zero cholesterol, low-fat meat alternative because of its chewy texture. In many recipes, you can veganize "chicken" recipes by substituting wheat meat or seitan for the amount of dead chicken called for in the recipe. That is what I have done with the turnovers—it is a recipe from Pepperidge Farm for its puff pastry shells, but it assumed those who used it were meat eaters.

Living Among Meat Eaters: Rules of Thumb

- View meat eaters as blocked vegetarians and their reactions to you as their symptoms of being blocked. When something happens, tell yourself, "This is happening because meat eaters are blocked vegetarians. What shall I do? I have the choice to respond or not to respond."

- Be at peace with your vegetarianism and help others see that you are at peace with your diet.

- The closer the relationship (family, lover, roommate), the more likely that dietary differences will bear the burden of many nondietary conflicts.

- Nonvegetarians are perfectly happy eating vegan meals, as long as they are unaware that they are doing so.

- Be patient. Assume everyone can become unblocked.

- Assume your needs will not be met in any meat-eating context—airplanes, countries, hosts, restaurants. Always have a backup plan when eating out.

- Don't let any rudeness spoil your experiences. Respond to offensive behavior according to the rules of etiquette, courteously, and move on.

- You have the right not to answer questions you are asked and to stop a conversation that makes you feel uneasy. Order multiple copies of *Why Vegan?* and *Vegetarian Living* and *101 Reasons I'm a Vegetarian,* and offer them to people who have questions for you.

- Don't talk about your vegetarianism at a meal if people are eating meat.

- Volunteer to bring something whenever you are invited somewhere.

- Get involved. Join a vegetarian society.

- Avoid dining out with your meat-eating friends when you are first converting.

- Don't let anyone coerce you into eating something you don't feel good about eating.

- Tell your friends that it is important to you to be a vegetarian and ask that they help you.

- Know that, even if you are the only one, you are doing the right thing.

- If offered meat, say "No thank you."

APPENDIX B

Letter to Parents of Vegetarians

Dear Parents,

The adolescent and preadolescent years of your children are a very special—and unusual—time. They transform your offspring from dependent child to autonomous adult. These are years of exploration and, by necessity, of rebellion. Your children must decide for themselves which of their childhood values are good and worthy of being held on to, and which of their childhood presumptions need to be examined and challenged. This is a very dramatic process! And now added to this volatile mix is vegetarianism!

Let me assist you in responding to their vegetarianism.

With adolescents, it is hard to know what is *your* issue and what is *their* issue; what you absolutely have to step on and redirect and what you need to leave alone. A wise counselor advised me in regard to my own two children (eleven and sixteen): "Hands off as much as possible." We have to allow our children to experiment and grow. We have to allow them to make wrong choices so that they learn the process of making good choices.

I once read an analysis of the fairy tale "Sleeping Beauty" that I found immensely helpful in relating to my own children. After Sleeping Beauty pricks her finger on the spinning wheel and falls into a deep sleep, vines with thorns grow all around the wall of the town. The thorns represent the difficult moods and reactions of the adolescent as he or she separates from the parents and becomes an adult. Just as, after time, the thorn vines become roses, so will our adolescents awaken from their adolescence and be in full bloom as adults. Whenever I feel particularly frustrated and rebuffed by my teenager, I remember that "this is his thorny period" and try to relax into this stage.

For you, the vegetarianism of your teenager may feel like those thorns. They keep you away from your child. They are a barrier, and a prickly one! But imagine that your child's vegetarianism is the beginning of the blossoming of adult values. After all, your children are not rejecting your values. They are manifesting a level of sensitivity and tenderness toward the feelings of living creatures. You must be the people who shaped these values.

An adolescent vacillates between separation and neediness. Their vegetarianism incorporates both ends of this continuum. They establish a separate identity through their vegetarianism, but they still have a neediness to be loved by you, accepted in who they are becoming. If you hear your child say, "If you really loved me, you would . . . [watch this video, stop eating meat, take me to those animal rights meetings . . .]" you are hearing the voice of an adolescent who is separating but still needy, connected to you but also distressed by a very alienating outside world. Don't get defensive; instead, assure them of your love. They are saying, "I am needy in this area, I need your love. I need your support." You can say, "We love you. You are changing. We will support you as you change, but that may not mean that we also change."

Remember that a judgmental tone is an aspect of adolescence. The tone and shouting is the way teenagers try to equalize the power between themselves and their very powerful parents. We may feel impatient or furious when a teenager announces an ultimatum, dismisses our concerns, or uses a tone of disdain in speaking with us, especially when challenging something we hold special. But be careful with your feelings. Even when we feel frustrated with them, we know that adolescents' tone of voice or shouting doesn't actually equalize power. So don't become susceptible to their thorns. Remember they are growing inside. Speak to them calmly and evenly. *Listen.* Ask them, "What are you feeling?" Always let them know you will listen.

Even if your adolescent wants you to take their diet personally, as a reproach of what you are doing, you don't need to interpret it that way.

Don't isolate them emotionally because a part of their anger is now turned toward you. It probably is turned toward their meat-eating peers as well. Indeed, when it comes to your children's vegetarianism, it is probably safe to assume that their friends and you—often on different sides of arguments—eerily agree. What does this mean for your children? They need you even more.

Don't tell them this is a phase that they'll outgrow, even if you think it is. This tells them you see them as being childlike. They want to be respected, not patronized. Don't treat it as a fad or simply as teenage rebelliousness. And don't discuss it with your friends in your child's presence. One mother scoffed at it as an experiment, and reported it derogatorily to her neighbor. Her daughter told me, "The worst is when she says 'It's just a fad' to her friends. I feel very bad."

Your kids are emulating the ideas of thinkers such as Gandhi and Thoreau. Praise them for taking an ethical stand. Ask your children to tell you the process they went through in deciding to become a vegetarian, and don't feel that they are judging you in their statements. And don't force them to eat meat. Don't tell them, "Well, just pick the meat out." Respecting them, even in their disagreements with you, teaches them the lesson of respect. You will discover this lesson blossoming in their lives in many ways. They will have learned it from you.

Of course you are worried about your children's nutritional needs. Your children can be perfectly healthy on a vegetarian or a vegan diet. Vegetarian children will reach the right height and weight for their age group. If they aren't eating well as vegetarians, they probably weren't eating well as meat eaters either. In fact, not only can a vegetarian diet be appropriate for any age group but vegetarians' diet may adhere more closely to the current dietary guidelines than that of nonvegetarians'. One teenager said to me, "Parents are always complaining that their kids aren't eating vegetables, and then when they eat only vegetables, they get upset." Use this as an opportunity to introduce them to foods you always wanted them to eat. Now you can say, "Look, a broccoli [chard, kale, spinach] casserole," and they may well be thrilled. The opportunities are endless!

If you feel vegetarianism is masking an eating disorder, these are the things to be alert to:

- If your child has continued to lose weight after being a vegetarian for two or three months. At first, the weight loss can be attributed to a number of factors (for instance, the move from a high-fat diet) and the time it takes to learn how to create healthy vegetarian meals. But after two or three months, weight loss signals a possible problem.

- If your child starts to skip meals regularly or says that she isn't hungry.

- If vegetarian foods that appear to be high in calories or that have fat in them are avoided—tofu, meat substitutes, peanut butter, breads, and pastas.

- Compulsive counting of fat grams and calories.

- Weighing frequently or reports of feeling bloated when eating normal portions.

- Ritualistic behavior around food—in the way they eat (cutting everything into minuscule pieces) or in the inflexible manner in which they eat; eating only at a certain time.

- Obsessive-compulsive behavior.

- Distorted body image. She comments that she needs to lose weight or is fat when she's at a healthy weight or thin.

Adopting a vegetarian diet, in and of itself, should not be interpreted as an eating disorder.

You may be concerned that your children need some nutrient in meat, and you determine to make sure they get it by hiding meat foods in the food you prepare for them. Please don't do this! You teach your children that they can't trust you. At times when you feel anxious for them, remind yourself that there is nothing in meat that children can't get from some other food.

Identify the practical issues of their vegetarianism for your household without judging the vegetarianism itself. Have shopping and cooking responsibilities become more demanding? This is a wonderful opportunity to involve your children in kitchen responsibilities. It equips them for life on their own. But don't stop cooking for them now, if you have always prepared meals for them and if you will continue to cook for the others in the household. This will send a message of rejection to your children. Identify ways that your food can include a vegetarian component. Ask your children to help you develop a menu of foods your whole family can embrace. I have met a lot of parents who became vegetarians as they tried the food their children were eating. They discovered that they felt better. But no one is trying to rush you into anything!

Remember, Sleeping Beauty does awaken from her thorny period. Will vegetarianism continue in their lives when they reach the full blossoming of adulthood? Let them decide for themselves. By treating your children with respect, you model how one respects another despite a difference of opinion. That is a great gift.

APPENDIX C

The Vegetarian Patrons of Restaurants Card

Do you want more restaurants to serve delicious vegetarian food? You can tell them so with a "Vegetarian Patrons of Restaurants" card. Make multiple copies of the card that you find on the next page. Fold it so that it fits into your wallet or billfold. After eating at a restaurant, fill in your evaluation and your comments and hand the card to the restaurant manager or mail it to the restaurant later.

As you fill it out, you can remind yourself: "I am doing this for me. I had a great/terrible/mediocre/pleasant meal here and this is a way to acknowledge that. I am doing this for the restaurant. There are other vegetarians who might want to come here. This information helps them. I am doing this for other vegetarians; I want them to have as good an experience as possible when they come here."

..........Dear Restaurant Manager,

According to a National Restaurant Association Gallup Poll, 20% of American adults are likely or very likely to look for a restaurant that serves vegetarian items when they eat out. Over 33% are likely to order specific vegetarian items.

<u>Vegetarians</u> do not eat meat, poultry, fish or other sea animals, beef or chicken stocks, lard, or gelatin. <u>Vegans</u> are vegetarians who also avoid dairy products, eggs, and honey. The easiest way to meet the needs of all vegetarian patrons is to offer vegan items.

This form is provided by *Vegetarian Patrons of Restaurants*. I hope you will find it useful in meeting the needs of your vegetarian patrons.

The variety, taste, and appearance of your <u>Veg</u>etarian items are:

superb_____   okay_____   need improvement_____ .

Your selection of <u>Veg</u>an items is:

superb_____   okay_____   needs improvement_____ .

Please flip for Comments.

VPR
VEGETARIAN PATRONS OF RESTAURANTS

SERVING VEGETARIAN PATRONS AND RESTAURANTS NATIONWIDE THROUGH INFORMATIVE AND HELPFUL COMMUNICATIONS.

A project of the Vegetarian Foundation. For copies of this card and information on vegetarian living, see Carol J. Adams, *Living Among Meat Eaters* (Three Rivers Press).

Comments:

_____

_____

_____

_____

_____

International Vegetarian Card

International Vegetarian Card

Physicians Committee for Responsible Medicine
5100 Wisconsin Ave., Suite 404, Washington, DC 20016
(tel) 202-686-2210 · (fax) 202-686-2216 *www.pcrm.org*

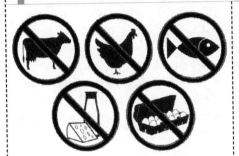

English	I'm a vegetarian. What do you recommend?
Arabic	آنا بكل خلاّر عش عناكم ؟
Czech	Jsem vegeterián/ka
Dutch	Ik beñ een vegetariër. Wat kunt U mij aanbevelen?
Finnish	Onko peillä kasvisrvokaa?

(continued on other side)

French	Je suis vegetarien(ne). Que me recommandez-vous?
German	Ich bin vegetarisch. Was empfehlen Sie mir?
Greek	Ειμαι χορτοφαγοσ. Τι μου προτεινετε.
Hungarian	Vegetáriánus vagyok, mit tudna ajánlani?
Indonesian	Saya tipak makan daging. Apa saran anda?
Italian	Sono un vegetariano/a. Cosa consiglia
Japanese	私は菜食主義です。 おすすめ料理は何ですか。
Malay	Saya tak makan danging. Apa yang anda cadangkan?
Maltese	Jien vegetarjan. X'tirrakommanda?
Mandarin	我吃素的 (I am a vegetarian.)
Norwegian	Jeg er vegetarianer. Hva vil du anbefale?
Philipino	Gulay lang ang kinakain ko. Ano ang maimumungkahi mo?
Portuguese	Eu son vegetariano/a. O que me aconselha?
Spanish	Yo soy vegetariano/a. ¿Que recomiende usted?
Swedish	Jag är vegetarian. Vad kan ni rekommendera?
Turkish	Ben veciteryanim. Ben et yemem.

Notes

p. ix. The epigraph to the book is from Mary Midgley, *Animals and Why They Matter* (Athens, Georgia: University of Georgia Press, 1983), p. 27.

p. 37. Erik H. Erikson, *Gandhi's Truth: On the Origins of Militant Nonviolence* (New York: W. W. Norton & Co., 1969), p. 142. (Language has been made inclusive.)

p. 53. The discussion of accusations on pp. 53–55 and "How very kind of them. I am deeply touched" draws upon Suzette Haden Elgin's *The Gentle Art of Verbal Self-Defense* (New York: Barnes and Noble, Inc., 1980, 1993), and specifically, p. 112.

p. 64. See my *The Inner Art of Vegetarianism Workbook* for exercises and tools that support the awareness, reflection, action model. The *Workbook* provides ways for blocked vegetarians to become unblocked.

p. 88. Sharon Salzberg, *Loving-Kindness: The Revolutionary Art of Happiness* (Boston and London: Shambhala, 1997), p. 52.

p. 104. Only 5 percent of all animals are killed by other animals. Ninety-five percent of all animals die from old age, sickness, exhaustion, hunger, thirst, changing climates, etc., and not by bloodshed. See Stephen Lackner, *Peaceable Nature: An Optimistic View of the Life on Earth* (New York: Harper & Row, 1984).

p. 116. The quotation from *The Sexual Politics of Meat: A Feminist-Vegetarian Critical Theory* (New York: Continuum, 2000) is found on pages 101–102.

p. 142. This is my variation of Suzette Elgin's analysis in *The Gentle Art of Verbal Self-Defense,* p. 66:

> "You don't care about 'X.'"
>
> "You *should* care about 'X.'"
>
> "You are rotten not to care about 'X.'"

Elgin's work is the base from which I have constructed my understanding of what is happening in verbal resistance tactics.

p. 172. Ken Haedrich, *Feeding the Healthy Vegetarian Family* (New York: Bantam, 1998), p. 152.

p. 175. "Chefs are not known for their small egos." Haedrich, *Feeding the Healthy Vegetarian Family,* p. 152.

p. 205. "Your friends who are world travelers and lovers of new experiences will be thrilled. . . ." Virginia and Mark Messina, *The Vegetarian Way.* New York: Crown Trade Paperbacks, 1996.

p. 216. Information on James Cameron's "Rose" draws from the obituary of Beatrice Wood by Roberta Smith in the *New York Times,* March 14, 1998.

p. 217. For the discussion of Joseph Campbell in *The Sexual Politics of Meat* see p. 201.

p. 217. Information on health costs for an individual's last year of life from the Robert Wood Johnson Foundation's website, summarizing A. A. Scitovsky, "'The High Cost of Dying' Revisited." *The Milbank Quarterly* 72, no. 4 (1994): 561–91. www.RWJF.ORG/Health/021577S.HTM

p. 303. "Your children are not rejecting your values. . . ." Paraphrase of an insight of Dr. Stanley Sapon.

p. 304. Information on identifying if vegetarianism is hiding an eating disorder is adapted from Ann Lien, "Vegetarian? Or Anorexic?" *Vegetarian Times,* September 1999, pp. 104–108.

Resources

Adams, Carol J. *The Inner Art of Vegetarianism.* New York: Lantern Books, 2000.
———. *The Inner Art of Vegetarianism Workbook.* New York: Lantern Books, 2001.
———. *The Sexual Politics of Meat: A Feminist-Vegetarian Critical Theory. Tenth Anniversary Edition.* New York: Continuum, 2000.
Beard, Christine H. *Become a Vegetarian in Five Easy Steps!* Ithaca, N.Y.: McBooks, Inc., 1997.
Boyd, Billy Ray. *For the Vegetarian in You.* Rocklin, Calif.: Prima Publishing, Inc., 1996.
Geon, Bryan. *Speaking Vegetarian: The Globetrotter's Guide to Ordering Meatless in 197 Countries.* Greenport, N. Y.: Pilot Books, 1999.
Havala, Suzanne. *The Complete Idiot's Guide to Being Vegetarian.* New York: Alpha Books, 1999.
Messina, Virginia and Mark. *The Vegetarian Way: Total Health for You and Your Family.* New York: Crown Trade Paperbacks, 1996.
Stepaniak, Joanne. *The Vegan Sourcebook.* Los Angeles: Lowell House, 1998.

COOKBOOKS

Bergeron, Ken. *Professional Vegetarian Cooking.* New York: John Wiley & Sons, Inc., 1999.
Bloodroot Collective. *The Perennial Political Palate: The Third Feminist Vegetarian Cookbook.* Bridgeport, Conn.: Sanguinaria Publishing, 1993.
Diamond, Marilyn. *The American Vegetarian Cookbook from the Fit for Life Kitchen.* New York: Warner Books, 1990.
Grogan, Bryanna Clark. *Nonna's Italian Kitchen: Delicious Home-Style Vegan Cuisine.* Summerton, Tenn.: Book Publishing Co., 1998.
Haedrich, Ken. *Feeding the Healthy Vegetarian Family.* New York: Bantam Books, 1998.
Hospodar, Miriam Kasin. *Heaven's Banquet: Vegetarian Cooking for Lifelong Health the Ayurveda Way.* New York: Dutton, 1999.
La Place, Viana. *Unplugged Kitchen: A Return to the Simple, Authentic Joys of Cooking.* New York: William Morrow and Co., 1996.
Madison, Deborah. *Vegetarian Cooking for Everyone.* New York: Broadway Books, 1997.

McCarty, Meredith. *Sweet and Natural: More Than 120 Naturally Sweet and Dairy-Free Desserts.* New York: St. Martin's Press, 1999.

Raymond, Jennifer. *The Peaceful Palate: Fine Vegetarian Cuisine.* Summerton, Tenn.: Book Publishing Co., 1996.

Stepaniak, Joanne. *Vegan Vittles.* Summerton, Tenn.: Book Publishing Co., 1996.

————. *The Saucy Vegetarian: Quick and Healthful No-Cook Sauces and Dressings.* Summerton, Tenn.: Book Publishing Co., 2000.

Tucker, Eric, and John Westerdahl. *The Millennium Cookbook.* Berkeley, Calif.: Ten Speed Press, 1998.

GROUPS

North American Vegetarian Society
P.O. Box 72
Dolgeville, NY 13329
518-568-7970
e-mail: navs@telenet.net

Physicians Committee for Responsible Medicine
5100 Wisconsin Avenue, N.W., Suite 404
Washington, DC 20016
202-686-2210
Web site: http://www.pcrm.org

The Vegetarian Resource Group
P.O. Box 1463
Baltimore, MD 21203
410-366-8343
Web site: http://www.vrg.org

Vegan Outreach
211 Indian Drive
Pittsburgh, PA 15328
412-968-0268
e-mail: info@vegliving.org
Web site: http://www.vegliving.org
Publishers of *Vegetarian Living* and *Why Vegan?* pamphlets

Vegan Action
P.O. Box 4288
Richmond, VA 23220
e-mail: info@vegan.org
Web site: http://www.vegan.org

Viva Vegie Society
P.O. Box 294
Prince Street Station
New York, NY 10012
646-424-9595
Publisher of Pamela Rice's *101 Reasons I'm a Vegetarian*

The Animals' Agenda
P.O. Box 25881
Baltimore, MD 21224
Web site: http://www.animalsagenda.org

United Poultry Concerns
P.O. Box 150
Machipongo, VA 23405
Web site: http://www.upc-online.org

Acknowledgments

I am thankful that I am part of a humane movement: one bite at a time, one meal at a time—we know all about the importance of seemingly small changes that are revolutionary in impact.

This book followed a visible and an invisible path.

Along the visible path, I benefited from those who reached out to embrace this project:

Pat Davis, who proposed the original idea out of which this book has grown, and who insisted that I not lose sight of the need for this book when I despaired of ever finishing it.

Patti Breitman, for saying yes to veganism and to me as a writer, for embracing this project early and waiting as I sorted it out.

The Kentucky Foundation for Women and Sallie Bingham for a week's residency at a women writer's retreat, where the book was begun.

Martin Rowe, for interviewing me about living among meat eaters for *Satya,* and printing my initial questionnaire. Martin's astute questions in that interview helped me sort out several of the most important themes in this book. Robin Armstrong, who posted my questionnaire at the newveg Web site and provided a form that could be answered through the Internet. Holly Lewis of vegetus.org, for permission to use the vegan lightbulb joke I found at her website.

Kim Stallwood for his support and *The Animals' Agenda,* for letting me explore this issue in the column "Living Among Meat Eaters," and specifically pages 61–62 and 162–164.

Vegans and vegetarians from around the world who e-mailed me and wrote to me about their experiences living among meat eaters in response to the *Satya* questionnaire or my online questionnaire. Thank you all so much, for taking the time to become a part of this book by answering my questions, sharing your despair, your frustrations, your commitments, your thoughts, and your joys. You have been living lives of abundance!

Gary Yousalvsky from ADAPTT, for a new way of describing what vegetarians don't eat.

Stanley and Rhoda Sapon, for their hospitality and insights.

My readers: Pat Davis, who plowed through several versions of some chapters, insisting on clarity. Steve Kaufman, for his careful reading of the manuscript, and for his many practical, insightful recommendations for improving it. Marie Fortune, for her wisdom on relationships. Mary Lou Randour, for suggestions, especially for her reflection on the role of guilt. Virginia Messina, for reviewing my letter to parents of vegetarians. Sarah Howery, whose vegetarianism prompted her mom to sug-

gest the need for this book and who, coming full circle, was my final reader, for her thoughtful responses.

Again, I am in the debt of the Richardson Public Library and its wonderful staff, especially the reference and Interlibrary Loan librarians, for finding books and information, and for their patience with my book-writing projects.

Kay Bushnell and Lynn Gale of the Vegetarian Foundation, for permission to reprint the "Vegetarian Patrons of Restaurants" card. It deservedly received a "Carrot" recognition from the *Vegetarian Times* in January 1995. I also thank Kay for creating wonderful nurturing recipes. Thanks to the good folks at Physicians Committee for Responsible Medicine, for developing the International Vegetarian Card and giving me permission to reproduce it in Appendix D. For his assistance in obtaining a copy of it, my thanks to Travis Moose of PCRM.

I am grateful for the attention to my ideas and the support of this book and me personally from the team of wonderful people at Three Rivers Press: Becky Cabaza, a jewel of an editor; Carrie Thornton, conscientious and caring; Anne Cherry, for prodding and pulling the correct words and syntax from me; Deborah Kerner for the beautiful design; and Brian Belfiglio, director of publicity, who has entered into the spirit of this book.

Vegetarian-cookbook authors give us all a great gift—the gift not only of creating great recipes, but taking the time to write them down, work with them, and experience the demands of publishing so that these recipes are shared with others. I am grateful for their generosity and creativity. I especially acknowledge Joanne Stepaniak, Jennifer Raymond, Ken Bergeron, and the women of the Bloodroot Collective, who run a feminist-vegetarian restaurant in Bridgeport, Connecticut, for permission to use their recipes. Authors of vegetarian cookbooks help each of us discover the abundance in the vegetarian choices we have made. Take the time to write a thank-you note to your favorite vegetarian-cookbook author.

Meat eaters who taught me so much about their fears, anxieties, and concerns about scarcity.

My invisible path, not conscious to me as I moved through it, was the path from scarcity to abundance. So many people and experiences touched me on this path. *The Inner Art of Vegetarianism* describes this path, which erupted from the pages of this book. Those who have nurtured me—friends and family—have nurtured within me this feeling of abundance. For friendship and love I thank: Pat Davis, Marie Fortune, Mary Hunt, Pamela Nelson, Christina Nakhoda, Carol Mai, Mary Lou Randour, my sisters, Nancy Adams and Jane Adams, and my parents, Muriel and Lee Towne Adams. The students around the country who brought me to their campuses, and introduced me to their ideas, their commitments, their recipes, have offered feelings of abundance as well. Martha Murphy Hall and Fred Dowd, who patiently teach coming home to this writer's body, reveal inner abundance to me.

And, as always, Bruce Buchanan, for living with, and loving so abundantly, this sometimes difficult, sometimes unrelenting, sometimes fragile, sometimes impulsive vegan. He has made this book and so much else possible.

Index

321

Looking for More Information?

Thank you for purchasing this book. I hope it was helpful and enables you to be the mover, not the moved, in this meat-eating world.

Have you had an experience living among meat eaters that you would like to share with me? I would love to hear from you. Contact me through my website: www.caroljadams.com. My website also explores the relationship between this book and *The Sexual Politics of Meat* and my other writings.

If you would like to reach me about lectures on the subject of living among meat eaters and my related topics, *The Sexual Politics of Meat* slide show and *The Inner Art of Vegetarianism* workshops, please contact me through my website.

I wish you the joy of abundance as you travel your vegetarian path.

About the Author

CAROL J. ADAMS is a nationally known writer and lecturer on the vegetarian lifestyle. Her landmark book, *The Sexual Politics of Meat,* was recently reissued on its tenth anniversary. She lives in Texas.